# A ROADMAP TO RECOVERY
## WRITTEN BY A VETERAN
## OF THE JOURNEY

Greg Anderson has devoted his life to helping cancer patients. Why? Because he realized that what *you* do after receiving a diagnosis of cancer makes a tremendous difference in the outcome of your illness and in the quality of your life each and every day. He understands that the initial response to hearing a diagnosis of cancer is fear and sometimes despair. He knows it is not the time to wade through a history of the disease or complicated medical texts. It is the time for quick, clear information and practical "action steps" to get you in control of your disease ... and your life. A compassionate, experienced cancer survivor, Greg Anderson offers specific help in deciding on the best course of treatment, on a lifestyle for health, and on achieving a positive attitude and inner peace. His book is packed with essential information, including self-quizzes, resources for support groups, the wisdom of dozens of cancer survivors, and lists for further readings. And best of all, it is from someone who received the diagnosis and made it a challenge to fight for life.

GREG ANDERSON, a survivor of lung cancer, is the bestselling author of two books, *The Triumphant Patient* and *The Cancer Conqueror*. He is founder and president of The Cancer Conquerors Foundation, a national educational and support organization committed to teaching patients and their families how to cope with cancer. He lives in Hershey, Pennsylvania, with his wife and family.

OTHER BOOKS BY GREG ANDERSON:

*THE CANCER CONQUEROR*

*THE TRIUMPHANT PATIENT*

# 50

## ESSENTIAL THINGS TO DO WHEN THE DOCTOR SAYS IT'S CANCER

### GREG ANDERSON

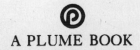

A PLUME BOOK

PLUME
Published by the Penguin Group
Penguin Books USA Inc., 375 Hudson Street, New York, New York 10014, U.S.A.
Penguin Books Ltd, 27 Wrights Lane, London W8 5TZ, England
Penguin Books Australia Ltd, Ringwood, Victoria, Australia
Penguin Books Canada Ltd, 10 Alcorn Avenue,
Toronto, Ontario, Canada M4V 3B2
Penguin Books (N.Z.) Ltd, 182–190 Wairau Road,
Auckland 10, New Zealand

Penguin Books Ltd, Registered Offices:
Harmondsworth, Middlesex, England

First published by Plume, an imprint of Dutton Signet,
a division of Penguin Books USA Inc.

First Printing, March, 1993
11   13   15   14   12

Copyright © Greg Anderson, 1993
All rights reserved

 REGISTERED TRADEMARK—MARCA REGISTRADA

LIBRARY OF CONGRESS CATALOGING IN PUBLICATION DATA:
Anderson, Greg
50 essential things to do when the doctor says it's cancer  |  Greg Anderson
p.  cm.
Includes bibliographical references.
ISBN 0-452-26954-7
1. Cancer—Popular works.   I. Title.   II. Title: Fifty essential
things to do when the doctor says it's cancer.
RC263.A617 1993                                        92–30902
616.99'4—dc20                                              CIP
Printed in the United States of America
Set in Caslon
Designed by Steven N. Stathakis

BOOKS ARE AVAILABLE AT QUANTITY DISCOUNTS WHEN USED TO PROMOTE PRODUCTS OR SERVICES. FOR INFORMATION PLEASE WRITE TO PREMIUM MARKETING DIVISION, PENGUIN BOOKS USA INC., 375 HUDSON STREET, NEW YORK, NEW YORK 10014.

*This book is dedicated to my wife, Linda, and our daughter, Erica.*
*Your unconditional loving sustains me.*

# ACKNOWLEDGMENTS

A heartfelt thank-you to all the friends of the Cancer Conquerors Foundation. I treasure you.

A very special thank-you to the New American Library family—especially Audrey LaFehr and Elaine Koster. I appreciate all you do and all you are.

To all who so generously gave their time, talents, and creativity to this project, please accept my sincere appreciation.

And to all who search these pages for the answers to wellness and to the world, my love.

# AUTHOR'S NOTE

The ideas in this book are meant to supplement the care and guidance of competent medical professionals. At no time does the author suggest that these steps take the place of conventional medical treatment. Do not attempt a self-diagnosis. Do not embark upon self-treatment of a serious illness without professional help. There are a growing number of doctors who will work with their clients. Find one. Form a healing partnership.

The characters in this book are composites of real people, but they are not intended to portray specific individuals.

# CONTENTS

# PREFACE

Patient empowerment, educating and motivating people to do all they possibly can to contribute actively to their health, has been the very cornerstone of my work for well over two decades. This book is a tribute to the spirit of patient empowerment.

I have seen hundreds of cases in which self-help has made the critical difference between life and almost certain death, between debilitating illness and robust health. The patient who proactively participates in his or her health care has a decided advantage. Truly we are fearfully and wonderfully made, with a capacity to help in our own healing.

This does not mean I advocate any approach to serious illness that excludes the best treatments conventional medicine has to offer. I am simply encouraging you to use *all* assets—your medical team, yourself, your mind, even your spirit. It is this combined approach that results in the best opportunity for your greater well-being.

The basic theme of *50 Essential Things to Do When the Doctor Says It's Cancer* is that every person must accept some of the responsibility for his or her own recovery. That idea is not new. But seldom has the call to help oneself been presented with more authority and conviction. Greg Anderson writes with intimate personal knowledge. In 1984, after being told he would die in thirty days, he set out to find patients who had lived after being told they were terminal. He hoped he could learn from them. Today Greg is not only alive, but his health is actually better than before this near-fatal experience.

There are never any guarantees in the world of medicine. But I would like to make one. If you practice the principles set forth in this powerful book, you will certainly increase your life quality. And that is often the first step to increasing your life quantity. This book articulates the concept of patient empowerment at its very best.

I wish you well.

KENNETH H. COOPER, M.D., M.P.H.
*The Cooper Clinic and Aerobics Center*
*Dallas, Texas*

# INTRODUCTION

*50 Essential Things to Do When the Doctor Says It's Cancer* is written for those people who want to survive the experience of cancer and who are willing to participate actively in the survival process. The book's goal is twofold: to help you clearly understand the prudent steps you can take after a cancer diagnosis; and to encourage you to take them.

This book is action-oriented, designed to help you put in motion a program that will maximize your opportunity for a complete recovery and an improved quality of life. This is not a book to be read and then put away, never to be looked at again. Treat it as your survival manual, something to refer to again and again. Turn to it to get "unstuck" in your cancer journey.

I believe this book has a meaningful message for every person affected by cancer. The principles are tailor-made for the person with a recent cancer diagnosis. If you or a loved one has recently been told, "It's cancer," you'll find right here the information you need to get control of your fears, analyze your diagnosis, and put in place the most effective treatment program possible. For the newly diagnosed, I recommend following the "50 Essential Things" in order. There is a certain logical progression in their sequence. Following this pattern will prove invaluable and will ensure that you are making the wisest decisions possible.

This book is also written for the person who has been diagnosed with a recurrence of cancer. Recurrence is a frightening event, a time of re-evaluation medically, emotionally, and spiritually. I encourage you to make the "50 Essential Things" the very heart of your entire analysis. Thoughtfully follow the steps. Use this book as your primary guide. A recurrence does not mean certain death. What you do *does* make a difference! See the "50 Essential Things" as mandatory points of action. Then you'll know you're doing everything you possibly can to contribute to your greater well-being.

This book is also for the "well" cancer patient. That description may seem like a contradiction in terms. It is not. Even those patients who enjoy remission or a complete recovery carry with them the lingering fear that cancer may strike again at any time. The "50 Essential Things" will give you the wellness principles you need to assure yourself that you are doing everything possible to retain your good health. Practice the principles. They are your best assurance of wellness on all levels.

Before you begin reading, get out a piece of paper and a pencil. I want you to create a wellness notebook. I started mine with a single sheet of my daughter's notebook paper and an old three-ring binder; nothing elaborate is required. As you read, questions and insights will come to mind. Write them down. You'll find yourself clipping newspaper and magazine articles about cancer. Put them in your notebook. This is going to become your primary source book, a reference manual for your personal cancer-recovery program. Now, nine years after I was told I would die, I have fourteen thick binders that house a wealth of insights and information important to me. And my notebook has also served as an excellent log that records my cancer journey.

Do the same. Even though the road map to recovery is contained in this book, each person must ultimately chart his or her own journey to wellness. Use your wellness notebook to record your unique personal insights. In particular, keep recording your questions. Then ask. Ask your doctor, your medical technicians, and other survivors. Nothing is to be assumed. Ask about medical terms that you don't understand. Ask about reasons for tests. Ask about the results of those tests. Ask for success stories. Ask. Ask. Ask. Asking questions gives you significant power. Do not be intimidated by the medical personnel or process. You are the one in charge. Ask!

Get started now. Take that next step. And always keep your hope alive!

GREG ANDERSON
*Fullerton, CA*
*January 1993*

# FOREWORD

For over twenty years, I have been working with an approach to cancer that includes the physical, mental, and spiritual. I have treated thousands of patients, with a relatively high rate of recovery, even from so-called "terminal" illnesses. I have learned a great deal about healing, and I have met some remarkable patients. Greg Anderson is one of them.

This book, *50 Essential Things to Do When the Doctor Says It's Cancer,* is a testimony to patients taking charge and choosing a stance of hope toward a diagnosis of cancer. Many of you who read this book are undoubtedly in a very difficult situation. Do not despair. Keep your hope alive. Learn from the experience of someone who was given a thirty-days-to-live prognosis. The author has been there. He knows what it's like to deal with the despair of cancer. He also knows what it's like to get well again.

While the road ahead may be difficult, I want you to know that it can be the most rewarding journey you will ever take. Even though the path through cancer requires work and discipline, it is also filled with discoveries that will excite and motivate you. Keep your focus on those joys.

Begin your journey now. Here, in this book, are the keys that can open the door for your return to good health. Take charge. Live this moment. Forgive. Love. You'll then know the power of hope. And you will be on the path to getting well again.

O. CARL SIMONTON, M.D.
*Founder, The Simonton Cancer Center*
*Pacific Palisades, CA*

# PART ONE

# ESSENTIAL UNDERSTANDING

# CHAPTER ONE

## WHAT'S HAPPENING?

### A DIFFERENT KIND OF ILLNESS

Cancer is the mutation of cellular genes resulting in the irregular growth of abnormal cells. The operative words here are *irregular* and *abnormal*.

Healthy cells of the body grow in predictable patterns. And as they wear out, they are replaced in an orderly manner by just the right number of new healthy cells.

Cancerous cells grow in an uncontrolled and unpredictable pattern. Their growth serves no useful biological purpose and often threatens the entire body. The cells themselves are mutant, changed in a way that limits their function. You have this condition in your body. Your cancer is one of more than one hundred cancers, each having its own site and other distinguishing characteristics.

Cancer is also a symptom of an inefficient immune system. Your understanding of this second point is of vital importance, critical in your decision to do all you can to help yourself get well. Your immune system is the first and most powerful defense your body has against cancer. For years you have periodically produced mutant cells that were potentially cancerous. In most cases the immune system was there to "clean up" the problems. Now it has not done so in an efficient enough manner to ensure your health.

This book will give specific steps to help you set in place a medical team and a treatment program in which you have confidence. The medical team and treatment program address the cellular portion of the illness. The book will also set out specific physical, psychological, and even spiritual action points that will enhance your greater well-being, enrich your life, and ultimately help you strengthen your immune system. These action points play an important role in mobilizing your powerful natural healing potential, your self-healing capabilities.

This is the body/mind/spirit connection. When used in conjunction with conventional medical care, this is the combination that gives you the greatest opportunity for survival. Your medical team will do all it can to remove or treat the mutant cells. Your task is to do all *you* can to enhance your immune system. Enhancing your immune system is done not so much by the doctor's medicine as it is by your own life-style choices. This means one's physical life-style, one's emotional life-style, and one's spiritual life-style.

The immune system is profoundly influenced by these choices. Tobacco use, improper diet, and lack of exercise are obvious deterrents to maximum immune function. So is mismanaged toxic stress, which fills the body with adrenaline and cortisone, both known to inhibit immune function.

Even your emotional reaction to the communication of the actual cancer diagnosis is a factor. The message "It's cancer" is received with great fear by most people. That fear can paralyze the recipient emotionally and psychologically at a time when intelligent action is required. And a spiritually toxic outlook after a cancer diagnosis can make a difficult situation a living hell. All of these responses have negative effects on immune function.

After putting your medical team in place, your concentrated efforts must be directed at your mind and spirit if you want to optimize your chances for survival. Fail to do so at your own peril. Retaining a medical team without doing all you can to help yourself is like attempting to walk with one stilt. It's possible, but the results are frequently disappointing.

The body/mind/spirit emphasis of this book and its principles should not cast doubts on the validity of scientific medicine. I do not encourage you to go back to the use of folk medicine, though I do have high respect for the old-fashioned family doctor. The only trouble with scientific medicine is that it is not scientific enough. In patient after patient we can observe the mind/body/spirit connection at work. But researchers cannot yet measure these obvious effects to their scientific satisfaction. Modern medicine will become truly scientific only when patients and their medical teams learn to manage the natural forces of the body, mind, and spirit within the context of a program for total recovery.

If you have cancer today, you can't wait for years of medical research to prove these points. This book will provide you with the most up-to-date body/mind/spirit knowledge available. Put these techniques to use in conjunction with the best that medicine has to offer. Therein lies optimum success.

Cancer is indeed a different kind of illness that demands a different kind of response. Recovery demands you and your participation. What you do *does* make a difference. For cancer patients who are determined to conquer this illness, that is very good news indeed.

## NO SUCH THING AS "HOPELESS"

You may have been told, "Get your affairs in order. You have a short time to live," or the favorite of the medical community, "Your illness is terminal." Don't believe it. Refuse to give in to that despair. Only God knows how long a person has to live.

In 1984 I was given a thirty-days-to-live prognosis. It was lung cancer. I had one lung removed. Four months later the cancer was back. This time it had invaded my lymph system. The surgeon put his hand on my shoulder and said, "The tiger is out of the cage. Your cancer is back. I'd give you about thirty days to live."

Part of the reason he was mistaken is that no surgeon can predict a patient's response to illness. After a couple of days of believing I would die, I made a profound decision. I decided to live!

By that I mean I made a decision to do all I could to triumph over the cancer. I determined to live each day I was given to the very best of my ability. I chose not to focus on the despair. I would adopt a stance of hopefulness. These decisions drastically changed my experience of illness. They resulted not only in better days but many more days as well. I believe such a decision may be able to do the same for you.

Some people, particularly those in the medical community, accuse me of spreading false hope. I believe there is no such thing. I believe there is only reasonable hope. And that is something that always leads to better days and perhaps more of them as well.

I deeply empathize with you and your medical condition. I have been there. I have been torn by the same emotions that now rip at you. I can identify with your fear and uncertainty. It is the most frightening time of your life.

Just remember, always choose hope. If you have been told that your time is limited, believe that life can still be a fulfilling adventure. Choose to live to the very fullest, discovering that every day is a good and perfect gift in spite of the circumstances. In that choice lies the seed of healing.

You *can* improve your chances for survival. What you do *does* make a difference. Choose hope. Dismiss despair. There is no such thing as a hopeless situation. Always choose and act on hope.

# CHAPTER TWO

## A
## ROAD
## MAP
## TO
## RECOVERY

### LEARNING FROM CANCER SURVIVORS

After my surgeon told me I had thirty days to live, I was stunned. One moment I was in tears, the next I was enraged. I thought it was all a mistake, convinced my tests had been confused with another patient's. I was filled with fear and self-pity. One afternoon I yelled out in anger, "Oh God, what can I do?"

That question was answered. No, God didn't part the clouds and speak. I've always been skeptical of any such claims. But figuratively, the clouds were parted. I had the distinct impression that my task was to go search for survivors. I became aware that I needed to find people who were "supposed" to die but had lived. And once I found them, I was to learn from their success stories.

To date I have interviewed more than five hundred survivors of "terminal" cancer. These are the people who have been told the equivalent of, "Get your affairs in order." These are the brave patients who, at one time, had no hope. These are the people whom the medical community gave up on.

But these people lived! These inspiring individuals, who possess no more courage or ability than you or I, shared some powerful lessons from which I was determined to learn. The principles on which they based their recoveries, and the action points, have worked for me and for thousands of other cancer patients. I believe the lessons can be pivotal in your life too.

After I conducted more than a hundred interviews, it became clear there were similar patterns to most of the individual stories. For example, the vast majority of survivors do not believe they got well by chance. The triumphant patients believe they worked for their wellness, earning it on a daily basis. Neither do most survivors credit their doctors alone for their recovery. Instead, the exceptional patients focus on mobilizing body, mind, and spirit in their quest for high-level wellness.

Pattern after pattern emerged from the survivor interviews. In 1988 I first summarized the principles and combined them into a simple plan that anyone could understand and put to use. The plan has since been refined by hundreds of additional interviews. Today, through the Cancer Survival Training programs of the Cancer Conquerors Foundation, tens of thousands of cancer patients have used these principles as a road map, a strategic plan, to enhance their health and enrich their lives.


## THE PRINCIPLES

Before we come to the "50 Essential Things," I'd like to go over the eight basic principles that cancer survivors have in common. The following categories emerged from the survivor interviews:

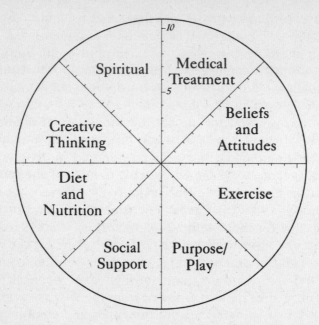

*Rate Yourself: After reading and studying each of the eight basic principles, return to this diagram and give yourself a rating for each category. 10=highest, 1=lowest. What does this tell you about your wellness and about your cancer journey? Take a break from your reading and consider the implications of this analysis.*

## PRINCIPLE #1: MEDICAL TREATMENT

The vast majority of cancer survivors start and complete a treatment program centered around conventional medical care. Surgery, chemotherapy/hormonal therapy, and radiation—often in combination—are the treatments of choice.

These forms of treatment are the conventional methods. This both surprised and encouraged me. I thought I might find survivors using nontraditional methods like exotic diets and "secret" potions. Yes, there were some who subscribed to such unconventional approaches. But the vast majority, more than

95 percent, adopted a medical plan of recognized and approved treatment.

It is important to note, however, that survivors do not just submit themselves to doctors for treatment. As you study the "50 Essential Things," you'll see how survivors actually take charge of the management of their entire medical programs. Survivors choose doctors in whom they have confidence and treatment programs about which they have convictions. Survivors are active patients, involved with each decision, making certain that they are fully informed and understand each option.

This idea of taking charge of one's medical program is the single most common practice among survivors. It is the cornerstone of a strategic recovery plan.

## PRINCIPLE #2: BELIEFS AND ATTITUDES

Cancer survivors choose beliefs and attitudes about their illness that serve them well. The most basic belief is that *cancer does not equate with death*. It is sad but true that much of the world still considers cancer and death to be synonymous. Not so with survivors.

Yet the majority of survivors are not "be-positive-against-all-evidence" sort of people. They have a refreshing sense of skepticism about "just-be-positive" solutions. Survivors are tough-minded realists, people who clearly understand what cancer may mean to their lives. Very few survivors have an attitude that says, "No problem. I'm fine. Everything's going to be all right." That's denial.

Instead, survivors recognize the truth—that their cancer may or may not mean death. This stance carries a vastly different outlook than either the superpositive or hopelessly negative. Survivors believe, "Yes, I may die. But I also may live. And I am going to invest my time, whatever its length, in living the best way I know how." Even those with the worst prognoses choose this belief first. Survival follows.

Survivors also hold unique beliefs about their medical treatment. Survivors challenge the conventional thinking about the effectiveness of their treatment and the treatment's potential side effects. They see their treatment as effective. They believe they will have minimal and manageable side effects. The "50 Essential Things" will help you understand and apply these key beliefs and attitudes toward your own treatment program.

You will probably not be surprised to learn that survivors hold another key belief about their role in illness recovery. They believe their active personal involvement is absolutely essential to the recovery process. Survivors believe wellness is no accident, that it takes work, and that it is their personal responsibility to make getting well the number-one priority in their lives. For the moment, getting well takes precedence over everything. Survivors believe that what they do makes a significant difference.

These powerful beliefs and attitudes help focus the efforts of survivors. Many survivors feel that positive beliefs and attitudes themselves have a biochemical reality that enhances healing. You'll recognize these beliefs and attitudes throughout the "50 Essential Things."

### PRINCIPLE #3: EXERCISE

Cancer survivors believe strongly in the importance of exercise. Nearly every person I interviewed emphasized the need for physical activity. There were swimmers, bikers, and lots of walkers. But most surprising were those patients who had been confined to hospital beds or wheelchairs, or who were otherwise physically limited. They would do full-body stretches in their beds, lift weights from their chairs, and do everything possible to honor their physical needs. It was inspiring to hear some of their stories.

I was moved to look at my own exercise habits early in my cancer journey. Second only to developing a belief that recovery was possible, I credit exercise with starting me on the path to recovery. It was not easy. I was weak and emaciated, at the point of lowest energy. But I started with stretching exercises, doing arm circles just until I felt an increase in energy. Then I added a walking routine, being certain to follow the increase-in-energy guidelines you'll find in the forthcoming pages. Soon I understood firsthand what other survivors had been telling me: "You've got to take charge of your body and command your body to move."

You'll come to see that exercise you enjoy is an important part of your own journey through cancer.

### PRINCIPLE #4: PURPOSE/PLAY BALANCE

Survivors feel wanted. They perceive a purpose for living, and they balance this purpose with activities that bring them joy. This is a major recurring theme among the community of cancer survivors.

The feeling of being needed and wanted expresses itself in many ways. Service to others is a consistent theme. Family is a major reason: "They couldn't get along without me." Important accomplishments or life milestones also enrich the life purpose for many survivors: "I determined I was going to celebrate my daughter's wedding." Importantly, most survivors are able to separate being needed from being unduly depended upon. Few are rescuers or feel forced to serve. Instead, they feel that they are privileged to be able to help others in meaningful ways. And in helping others, they help themselves, thus reinforcing the perception they are wanted and needed.

Survivors balance purpose with play. Survivors often abandon themselves to just having fun. Hobbies of all sorts bring joy to this extraordinary group. I am struck by the large number who enjoy gardening, both flowers and vegetables. Male, female, city, or rural, it doesn't seem to make much difference. Many survivors express deep satisfaction in seeing their efforts produce new life. I sense that the growing plants serve as a metaphor for their own physical and spiritual journeys through cancer and through life.

Purpose/play balance provides an integration of normalcy into survivors' lives when they could easily become over- whelmed by the fear and despair of cancer.

## PRINCIPLE #5: SOCIAL SUPPORT

Relationships. Cancer survivors give more time and energy to relationships that nurture them and invest themselves less in relationships that are toxic. This may seem like a benign prac- tice, but it has some surprising implications that survivors be- lieve are central to their being alive.

Good relationships with friends, relatives, lovers, spouses, children, employers, co-workers, employees—or the lack of them—build us up or tear us down. Survivors are "relationship sensitive," examining, perhaps for the first time in their lives, how they get along with other people. It is common for survi- vors to put relationships "on hold," especially during the medical-treatment process. This doesn't mean survivors auto- matically kick "toxic" people out of their lives for all time. But it certainly means a reduced emotional investment in those re- lationships.

Cancer also gives patients permission to examine their vo- cational relationships. The same is true of friends and family. Survivors actively examine their entire social-support structure. Changes often follow. Much of the actual work of getting well again takes place within this arena.

Social support extends to support groups. Cancer survivors know the importance of mutual aid, having practiced it long be- fore support groups became fashionable. Today the prolifera- tion of cancer support groups makes this service within the reach of any person who desires to attend. Survivors make sup- port groups part of their recovery process.

## PRINCIPLE #6: DIET AND NUTRITION

Cancer survivors make significant diet and nutritional changes. Among survivors there is an almost universal recognition of the important contribution diet makes to recovery. However, there is anything but universal agreement on what those changes should be.

Survivors eat with awareness. They stop feeding themselves for emotional and psychological reasons and commit to fueling their bodies for physical reasons. Survivors eat premium foods that are low on the food chain. Fresh fruits, fresh vegetables, and whole grains are their new foods of choice. A marked decrease in meat, particularly red meat, is found among survivors. Many adopt vegetarian practices.

While vitamin and mineral supplementation is widely practiced among survivors, there exists a great diversity in actual practices. Some survivors use many supplements extensively, while others settle for a daily multiple vitamin.

I can report no consensus in the arena of diet and nutrition except for attitude. While nutritional practices vary, survivors do agree on one thing: They have an excited belief that nutrition is another thing they "get" to do to get well again. This attitude is very important.

## PRINCIPLE #7: CREATIVE THINKING

Survivors use the mind to heal. Affirmations, meditation, and imagery are widely employed within the context of a comprehensive treatment program. Survivors use meditative techniques to reduce the symptoms of illness, manage the side effects of treatment, and improve emotional well-being.

I am struck by how many survivors use affirmations to manage their emotions. Our culture tells us that positive feelings are desirable and negative feelings are not. Survivors have a more accurate way of looking at emotions. They seem to accept whatever emotions they have, be they positive or negative, as okay. Survivors tend to be realists who recognize that the cancer journey has tremendous emotional hills and valleys. So they accept the emotions that accompany these roller-coaster feelings.

But survivors do not get stuck in those feelings. They are able to rise above negative emotions by using their minds to focus positively on living in the moment. Survivors use affirmations, often a simple phrase or verse, to gain emotional comfort and control rather than allowing runaway feelings to rule their lives.

The "50 Essential Things" will detail several of these and help you implement them in your own recovery program. For survivors, the mind is another powerful resource to mobilize in the getting-well journey.

### PRINCIPLE #8: SPIRITUALITY

Survivors develop a more spiritual outlook in their lives. They see life differently than prior to their brush with death. While many cancer patients focus on a body that may be riddled with disease or mourn over dreams that are hopelessly derailed, survivors tend to see the high value of what is simple and readily available in life in spite of their illness.

A more spiritual outlook is not necessarily an issue of religion; many survivors eschew traditional religious practices that emphasize doctrines and creeds. The brand of spirituality you see in cancer survivors is not some sweet platitude from the past. For many survivors it is a radical although serene response to the world. Experiencing inner peace is the goal. Survivors find there is much healing in this pursuit.

## IMPLEMENTATION INTELLIGENCE

Each of the eight principles is important, but they are not always equal. For example, the timing is different. At the time of the initial diagnosis, nearly all the emphasis may be placed on medical treatment. This is appropriate. After the treatment program is in place, survivors may then place more emphasis on beliefs and attitudes or diet and nutrition. Only later may they begin the work of social support or focus on another principle.

Each survivor creates his or her own plan within the structure of these eight principles. One principle takes priority at the appropriate time. Seldom do survivors make simultaneous wholesale changes in all eight areas. Those who tried to change too much too quickly often met with temporary defeat and had to start again.

But each principle has its place in the recovery program of most cancer patients. Even though there is a difference in timing, many survivors note, in retrospect, that resolving a relationship problem may have been just as important in their recovery as medical treatment! The "live" signals that proper diet and exercise give to the body are so strong that many survivors rate diet and exercise on a par with or even above the contribution of traditional medicine to their getting well. But nearly all survivors agreed it was the *balance*, the comprehensive approach that included, but did not stop at, conventional medicine, that made recovery possible. Survivors also felt they *earned* their health back but at the same time stood in awe of the body's immense natural power to heal itself.

The eight principles create the strategic framework for cancer patients to follow in their recovery process. The strategic plan is the context in which the "50 Essential Things" are implemented. The circle is the map. The 50 things are the steps survivors take while consulting the map.

# PART TWO

---

# THE
# 50
# ESSENTIAL
# THINGS
# TO DO

# Chapter Three

## Determining Your Treatment Program

Your top priority following a cancer diagnosis is to put in place the best medical treatment program you can possibly obtain. But this is not as simple as going to one doctor and saying, "Treat me."

The decisions you make authorizing your cancer-treatment program are some of the most important decisions you will make in your entire life. Begin the journey through cancer by following a course of action that has proven highly successful for thousands of cancer survivors.

# #1

# STOP
# "AWFULIZING"

You've been told, "It's cancer." I have deep compassion for you and fully appreciate your feelings. First, you're in shock and filled with fear. The next moment you're angry but not quite certain at whom. Then comes the guilt and thoughts of "Did I bring this on myself?" Plus all the questions that have started to rush through your mind: "Will I die?" "How long do I have?" "What will happen to my family?" And on and on and on. Your mind is overwhelmed at times.

Be calm. Try not to panic. I know that this is easier said than done for many people, but be aware that panic will only get in the way of rational and positive action.

Cancer is a serious illness but *it is not necessarily fatal*. You do have the luxury of some time. Unlike a heart attack or a severed artery, cancer does not require you to do something this very instant. Don't take that as license for inaction. But be aware that an immediate response, often based in fear and panic, is not only *not* required, it may be harmful.

Stop and examine your frenzied thoughts for just a moment. It is at the beginning stages that clear decision making will be most important, to ensure that your illness is properly treated. Uncontrolled panic acts only to your detriment.

Panic is an issue of the mind, of our thoughts about cancer, and can accurately be labeled as *awfulizing*. Isn't that an apt description? In our minds we take our current situation to its worst possible conclusion.

If we can observe our emotions objectively just for a moment, we will see something different. The intense panic that virtually every cancer patient experiences is actually the mind projecting its fears into the future. Think of that. *Panic is a projection that is not real.* We are not just our fears. Our fears do not necessarily determine our future. This is significant.

What to do? When you start to feel anxious emotions arising inside, try to witness them. Just observe. See them and yourself in your mind's eye. Instead of putting yourself in the role of a victim who is hopelessly caught in a web of despair, become the observer. By not engaging the mind in battle, by simply watching and letting go, your emotions will soon become quiet.

Then imagine yourself as an effective problem solver, a person who is about to make some very important choices. Clear decision making can be yours.

### AN IMPORTANT THING YOU CAN DO

Sit down. Take a deep breath. Say out loud, "Cancer does not mean death." Observe your emotions. Detach by separating who you are as a person from the emotional panic you may be feeling. You are not uncontrolled panic even though you may be *experiencing* panic. The two are very different. Read and act on the next two steps in this book.

# #2

---

# TAKE
# CHARGE

Who is the most important person on your team? Some people believe it is their surgeon. Others believe it is their oncologist. Some choose the medical technicians, others the nurse, and still others choose their spouse.

But the most important person on your wellness team is you! You are the one who is ill. It is you who must work to get well again. You are the central character. You are in charge.

Too often patients surrender leadership. Elizabeth was a thirty-eight-year-old housewife who had been diagnosed with metastatic breast cancer. Her treatment was not going well, which left Elizabeth discouraged. Her doctor kept assuring her, "We're doing all we can. Trust me."

One day Elizabeth said to herself, "Do I accept the course of this treatment or do I try something else?" She called and made an appointment at a Clinical Cancer Center that was a four-hour drive from her home. Doctors there recommended a different treatment program that Elizabeth took back to her home doctor for implementation. "Personally taking charge was my turning point," explained a healthy Elizabeth four years after her bold decision.

See yourself as the manager of a baseball team, or whatever organizational analogy you like, whose task it is to get you well. You'll want a strong starting pitcher; many times that is the doctor. And you'll need many other team members: a catcher, infielders, outfielders. Equate these with specialists, technicians, family, friends, and support groups. And you are the manager, choosing the team that is on the field at any given time.

This is a big hurdle to many patients. It's a learned attitude. Traditionally, consumers play a passive role in the health care system, going along with whatever doctors and hospitals recommend. We're encouraged to consent to rather than challenge recommendations. This passive attitude will not do. Decide to take charge now!

### AN IMPORTANT THING YOU CAN DO

Evaluate your team. Who is managing this team? Who are the players? Is it a one-person show, when many more people could be helping? Are the team members working for you or do some seem to be working against you? One woman remarked, "Every time I go to the doctor, I feel like I am in enemy territory." If you feel that way, it may be a signal that you need to make a substitution. Remember: You are the person in charge!

# #3

## ASK
## YOUR
## DOCTOR
## THESE
## QUESTIONS

It is very important for you to clearly understand your diagnosis. The doctor who diagnosed you needs to answer the following questions. You need to *write down* the answers:

1. Precisely what type of cancer do I have?_____

_____

2. Has it spread beyond the primary site? If so, where?_____
3. How did you determine this diagnosis?_____

_____

4. Is there any indication that a second pathology report is needed?_____

5. Are you recommending additional tests? What are you looking for with each test?_____

_____

6. How certain are you that my tests and the resulting diagnosis are accurate?_____

7. What are my treatment options? Which one(s) do you recommend?_____

_____

8. Will you obtain and review with me the information on my type and stage of cancer from the National Cancer Institute's Physicians Data Query (PDQ) program?_____

9. Whom would you recommend for a second opinion?\_\_\_\_\_

10. Are you a board-certified oncologist?_____

As a cancer patient you are a consumer. The decision process regarding who will prescribe and administer your treatment is not that much different from any other major purchase decision. But the consequences of your decisions are radically different from those involved in buying an automobile, for example. You have the right, even the responsibility, to ask questions of your doctor just as you would with any consumer purchase. Evaluate those answers more closely than any major purchase you have ever made. Your options and choices for the best treatment will then become clear.

Cancer survivors are consumer activists. They ask. Become an activist!

### AN IMPORTANT THING YOU CAN DO

Get the preceding questions answered today! Record the answers in your wellness notebook. Ask them again when you seek your second opinion.

# #4

# GET
# A SECOND
# OPINION

Get a second opinion from a board-certified oncologist, a cancer specialist. If at all possible, this should be done prior to starting any treatment.

The second opinion should come from a doctor in a different medical group from the first, even from a separate hospital. Ask the doctor who made the initial diagnosis for a complete transcript of your records. Take the records with you or have them sent ahead.

"I had a second opinion all right," explained Katherine, a fifty-five-year-old insurance-office manager and grandmother, describing her experience with breast cancer. "The second opinion came from another surgeon who shared offices with the first. They both said a radical (mastectomy) was the way to go. And to this day I wonder if I would have been better off with a lumpectomy and radiation."

Katherine's second-opinion experience could have been improved in two ways. First, she would have been better served by consulting with an oncologist. These specialists diagnose and treat cancer every working day. They can be expected to have the most up-to-date information on treatment options for each type and stage of cancer. Both surgeons Katherine talked to were located just down the hall from her family doctor. They were general surgeons who dealt with a variety of illnesses, not just cancer.

Second, Katherine would have been better served by consulting with a second-opinion doctor not associated with the first. These associations are a little-discussed but potentially important issue to patients. Doctors who are friends, office mates, business associates, or in a junior position within a medical practice may find it difficult to challenge the diagnoses or recommended treatment programs of associates. All sorts of relationships exist that may influence decisions. "We were in the middle of renegotiating the lease," said Robert, a young oncologist who rented office space from another oncologist. "We were meeting that very afternoon to discuss rents. I didn't want to offend my landlord when he sent me a patient for a second-opinion consultation. So I just agreed with his treatment recommendations."

That experience may seem improbable, but the story is unfortunately true. The best safeguard is to seek a second opinion from a board-certified oncologist who is in a different practice, a different hospital, perhaps even a different city, than the doctor making the initial diagnosis.

One of the very best places to get a second opinion is from a National Cancer Institute–designated Comprehensive Cancer Center or a Clinical Cancer Center. If those centers are simply too far away from your home, hospitals involved in the Community Clinical Oncology Program might be your next choice. Contact the Cancer Information Service, referred to in the next step, to find the location nearest you.

Getting a second opinion in no way implies that the initial diagnosis is incorrect or that the suggested treatment is inappropriate. On a subject as important as this, you simply deserve to have the benefit of more than one person's thinking. Your second-opinion search also puts you in touch with other doctors, helping you decide which medical team will actually administer your treatment program.

John was a sixty-two-year-old diagnosed with colon cancer, who was consulting with a surgeon as his primary treatment provider. The day John's second set of test results came back, the doctor called him, confirmed the initial diagnosis and said, "You're scheduled for surgery at 2:00 tomorrow afternoon. Be at the hospital by 8:30 tomorrow morning." Fortunately, John had the courage to say "slow down" and went about getting a second opinion from a qualified oncologist.

The second-opinion oncologist independently confirmed the initial diagnosis. In fact, he also recommended surgery, just as John was initially advised. So John returned to his surgeon only to be greeted with sarcasm: "I told you so. What's the matter? Didn't you trust me?" John walked out of that doctor's office, found another surgeon, and today is doing fine.

### AN IMPORTANT THING YOU CAN DO

Make your appointment for a second opinion *today*. This is one of the most important things you can do. Do not overlook this step. Act on this now!

# #5

## MAKE
## AN IMPORTANT
## PHONE
## CALL

You have an important ally just a phone call away. In the United States dial 1-800-4-CANCER. This will put you in touch with a trained staff member of the National Cancer Institute's Cancer Information Service (CIS). All inquiries are treated confidentially. There is no charge.

CIS is designed to give you up-to-date, accurate, and understandable information and facts about your type of cancer. Have them send you information on your specific type of cancer, the most important information being the state-of-the-art treatment options for your type and stage of cancer.

If you are dealing with a cancer that the doctors say will not respond to conventional treatment, ask the CIS staff member to access the PDQ (Physicians Data Query) service for information on current experimental therapies.

AN IMPORTANT THING YOU CAN DO

Call 1-800-4-CANCER today. Become informed!

# #6

## RETHINK
## THE
## STATISTICS

Nick, who has lung cancer, accurately expresses most patients' feelings about cancer statistics: "When I look at those numbers, I get scared to death."

You will soon hear and read cancer-recovery statistics that detail cancer incidence, mortality, and five-year survival rates. Do not let these statistics paralyze you. Your response to them is critical.

Statistics measure populations. And they can be interpreted in a great many ways. But statistics do not determine any individual case, including yours.

Just after my second surgery, I received a booklet filled with numerical tables, statistics, and graphs on all types of cancers. Of course I felt compelled to read all the information. The numbers on metastatic lung cancer were not promising. As I reflected on what I read, I felt frightened, depressed, and filled with despair, certain of my fast-approaching death.

Some days later I looked again at those statistics and realized that many people do survive. "What did they do?" I wondered. "How can I learn from them?"

No matter how difficult your situation, you must realize that there is no type of cancer that does not have some rate of survival. This is a significant fact. And it is cause for reasonable hope. The question now becomes, "What can I do to maximize my chances of getting on the right side of these statistics?"

With this book you have already begun to tap into the answers.

### AN IMPORTANT THING YOU CAN DO

Interpret statistics as indications of progress and hope. Determine to act with the conviction that hope is your greatest ally and that you will be counted as a "survivor statistic."

# #7

# UNDERSTAND
# YOUR
# TREATMENT
# OPTIONS

Your oncologist will explain which types of treatment might be used for your particular type and stage of cancer. These options will typically fall into one of three categories: surgery, chemotherapy/hormonal therapy, and radiation. A fourth category for cancers that are more advanced or those that simply do not respond to conventional treatment is investigative or experimental therapy.

Surgery is the most common form of cancer treatment. Surgical procedures are used to perform biopsies, remove malignant tumors, and relieve pain. Surgery is often the first phase of a more complete treatment program. For some types and stages of cancer, surgery will not be appropriate or even possible. If you are one who is told that your cancer is inoperable, do not despair. Recognize that *inoperable does not mean incurable!*

Your choice of surgeons is important. If your oncologist suggests surgery, the decision as to who actually performs the procedure is yours. You're more likely to get a well-qualified surgeon if you choose one who is a fellow of the American College of Surgeons and who is also board-certified in his or her field. Only about half of practicing surgeons are board-certified, so be sure to ask.

Chemotherapy is the treatment of cancer using chemicals. Hormone therapy is closely related to and often used in conjunction with chemotherapy. These drugs typically prevent cancer cells from rapidly reproducing or may actually destroy the cancer cells themselves. Chemotherapy/hormonal therapy may be in pill form and be taken by mouth, or it may be in liquid form and injected into a muscle or given through a vein or artery. The drugs may be administered in a daily, weekly, or monthly program for periods ranging from a few months to a lifetime in some cases.

Many cancers respond very well to chemical treatment. Side effects, once the fear of all patients, are now being more effectively controlled and vary widely from individual to individual. Refer in this book to #36, "Minimize Treatment Side Effects," for helpful things you can do to control unwanted side effects.

The administration of chemotherapy is an art, not an exact science. If your oncologist suggests chemotherapy or hormone treatment, ask about *chemo sensitivity testing*. Here, samples of your tissue are chemically analyzed in laboratory tests. This may help in establishing the most effective personalized treatment program before you begin. But be prepared for changes in the treatment program. It is common to try different chemotherapy drugs and different combinations of chemicals. These changes are the oncologist's attempt to improve the efficiency of the treatment.

Radiation therapy is the use of X-rays or gamma rays to damage the cancer cells so that they can no longer continue to divide and multiply. This therapy is most often administered by means of an external-beam machine. Internal radiation is becoming more common. Here, radioactive material is surgically implanted into or on the area to be treated. You will maximize your opportunity for receiving excellent care if you choose a physician who is certified by the American Board of Radiology.

Surgery, chemotherapy/hormonal therapy, and radiation therapy are the major "conventional" cancer-treatment options. They are the most proven and widely accepted treatment programs. Ask your oncologist what role each of these modalities may have in your case.

All cancers are treatable. Even in cases where the cancer is advanced, experimental investigative programs are available. If your cancer is not responding to conventional treatment, ask about biologic response modifiers, bone-marrow transplantations, and hyperthermia. You are entitled to understand the full range of treatments available. And from that understanding, you will have the knowledge and power to make the most intelligent treatment decisions.

In interviews with hundreds of cancer survivors, the overwhelming majority told me they started and completed a course of conventional therapy. It is a myth that cancer survivors turn to alternative, nontraditional cancer treatments in large numbers. In the late 1980s a Food and Drug Administration study estimated that as many as 40 percent of cancer patients used unconventional treatments. That may be true of the overall cancer population, although I doubt it. It is definitely *not* true of cancer survivors. The fact is, the vast majority of survivors select a conventional program using surgery, chemotherapy/ hormonal therapy, or radiation, often in combination, as the foundation of their treatment. The survivors then *supplement* this conventional program with many of the ideas presented in this book. I strongly recommend you do likewise. This combination represents your very best opportunity for surviving cancer today.

Contrary to myth, you do have several excellent cancer-treatment options open to you. You need to understand which one, or which combination of options, will best serve you. Make this determination in consultation with your board-certified oncologist and you will be sure that you are maximizing your recovery opportunities.

### AN IMPORTANT THING YOU CAN DO

Ask your oncologist to explain in depth the specific treatment options available to you in the areas of surgery, chemotherapy/hormonal therapy, and radiation. Ask for his or her recommendation. Record this information in your wellness notebook. But do not give your approval for treatment yet. There is more work to be done first.

# #8

# GAUGE
# YOUR
# CONFIDENCE
# IN YOUR
# DOCTOR

Few patients have any objective way to judge whether their surgeon, oncologist, or other medical professionals have technical competence. We can consider the experience of other patients and their doctors, but few of us can objectively or technically evaluate whether a particular doctor will be able to address our specific case with success. We can, however, make some nonobjective assessments, the kind of judgments that can be enormously important in any recovery journey: We can intuitively gauge our confidence level.

Ann is a successful career woman who developed ovarian cancer. By the time it was discovered, the metastasis was significant and the prognosis poor. Ann had no objective way to choose her treatment team.

Ann interviewed seven different oncologists. She came to them with her pathology report and diagnosis in hand and simply asked to talk to them for about twenty minutes. Her question was, "Assuming this diagnosis is correct, what would you have me do?"

The answers she received were actually fairly predictable and consistent. That was reassuring. But what was more reassuring was one oncologist's interpersonal skills. He asked questions to determine Ann's confidence in a procedure. And based on Ann's answers, and her confidence level, he offered his recommendations. Ann chose this doctor.

Ann's analysis was based not so much on any objective measures of technical competence but on her confidence, her belief in a person and his recommended program. She followed her intuition.

Know this: An excellent bedside manner can seldom make up for a lack of technical competence. But there is a direct correlation between the confidence one has in one's health care team and one's probability of recovery. And interpersonal skills shape that confidence level. You are seeking a balance here.

### AN IMPORTANT THING YOU CAN DO

Evaluate your confidence level following an encounter with your health care team. This is particularly important when you are being asked to make treatment decisions. If there is more doubt than assurance in your feelings toward the medical team and the treatment recommendations, it is time either to change your confidence level or change your team.

---

Be sure you are approaching this work at a comfortable pace. I suggest you take a break now and reflect on this important step. Continue your work after you have rested.

# #9

---

# CONVICTION
## VERSUS
# WISHFUL
# THINKING

Elaine had just been told by her doctor that an aggressive course of chemotherapy, one that would require hospitalization, was recommended.

Elaine was fearful of such a program. Still vivid in her memory was her mother-in-law's agonizing death from cancer, after going through a program of chemotherapy that seemed worse than the illness. Elaine vowed at that time that she would never have chemotherapy if she had cancer. Now she faced precisely the situation she most feared.

Elaine went in search of nontraditional treatments. Among others, she consulted a naturopath, who suggested a combination of herbs and hyperthermia, the use of heat, to help kill cancer cells. While this program sounded minimally toxic and noninvasive, Elaine now feared she was getting too far away from conventional medical care.

Then Elaine went to yet another medical oncologist. After she explained her fears and her research, this doctor recommended the use of hormones. Elaine was assured that hormonal therapy was typically less toxic than chemotherapy and in most cases generated far fewer side effects. But the hormone treatment was not as highly recommended as the original and more effective chemotherapy program.

Torn between these three different approaches, Elaine realized that the treatment she was most convinced would work was a combination of two. Through sheer persistence she was able to find an investigative technique that combined fractionated-dose chemotherapy with hyperthermia. And on her own she adopted a nutritional supplement program that included the herbs. She decided to hold the hormone treatment in reserve if she needed it.

Elaine's choice of treatment is clearly not the answer for everyone. But following one's conviction is an important element of every successful treatment program. Today, eleven years after her initial diagnosis, Elaine's cancer remains in remission, and she leads a full and happy life.

### AN IMPORTANT THING YOU CAN DO

Before you commit to a treatment program, take the time to ask a couple of questions: "Do I really hold the belief that this is the right thing to be doing?" "Or am I just taking the path of least resistance?" If you don't believe in it, *resist!* Find a program that has your conviction.

# #10

# REFLECT ON
# THE TREATMENT
# DECISION

If you've carefully read each step up to this point, you'll realize that you've simply been gathering information about treatment options and are not yet making any treatment decisions. Now it is time to systematically review your treatment options one last time prior to crossing this Rubicon.

First compare. Are you getting consistent information from:

- the doctor who made the initial diagnosis?
- the oncologist whom you consulted for your second opinion?
- the recommendations you received from your call to the Cancer Information Service?

You should expect to see a consistency in the recommendations you receive from these three sources. If there is agreement, your decision-making process will probably be straightforward.

If the recommendations of the doctors and the materials

from the Cancer Information Service are inconsistent, then your information gathering is not complete. When you receive mixed signals, it is a certain sign to *obtain a third qualified and independent opinion*. Believe me, this is time and money wisely spent.

Many people in the medical community scoff at such a suggestion. The objections are predictable: "You're wasting valuable time that could be spent treating the disease." Or a more benign comment: "The differences in treatment that you'll find are actually very minor." I disagree.

In all but the very rare case, the few days spent in gaining a third or fourth opinion are well worth the wait. As a patient you are after the very best treatment. You should expect a consistency of recommendations if not a consensus.

Terry is a forty-seven-year-old from Indiana who was diagnosed with lymphoma. He obtained *eight* different opinions before agreeing to a program of treatment. Terry's determination to find the best has proven wise, and today he is alive and well.

Terry's experience uncovers an objection patients often raise: "But my insurance won't cover a third opinion." My response is, "So what?" Mine didn't. I was only too glad to personally pay for the services of qualified medical experts who would help determine the best course of treatment for me. Develop a similar attitude. Don't let insurance coverage determine this issue. Borrow the money or seek out a free clinic. If you have received mixed signals, there is nothing more important in your life at this moment.

Once there is a clear choice for you to make in terms of medical treatment, a choice in which you have confidence, another evaluation needs a second reflective look. Are you comfortable with the people who will give you treatment and the place where the treatment will be administered?

June was a single mother in her fifties who had ovarian cancer. The treatment program in which she had the most confidence was recommended by doctors at a Comprehensive Cancer Center that was located more than an hour's commute on busy California freeways. She was expected to visit the center weekly while undergoing treatment. The commute was a problem for June. She didn't want to drive in rush-hour traffic. A friend or family member would have to act as chauffeur. And she didn't feel completely safe in the part of the city where the center was located.

June expressed her feelings about the drive and her physical safety to the supervising oncologist. The doctor's response was compassionate and understanding. He was able to make arrangements at a hospital only ten minutes from June's apartment. She could receive her weekly treatments there and visit the center just once a month. To this day, June believes the change in location was an important part of her successful recovery. This is another lesson in being assertive and asking.

Does the recommended treatment program truly have your conviction? Are you convinced that the recommendations are the very best? Conviction implies a sense of certainty. While there are no guarantees, your treatment program and the people who administer it should elicit a strong degree of certainty that this is the right path to be taking at this time.

I've helped hundreds of cancer patients walk through this treatment-option analysis. Invariably the question arises, "What about all the alternative approaches? I really haven't checked them out." I have consistently recommended this strategy: *First*, exhaust the conventional treatment options. Surgery, chemotherapy, and radiation are the basis for the vast majority of survivor success stories. If the conventional treatment methods hold no promise or are unsuccessful, *then* analyze both the investigative options, through National Cancer Institute–sponsored clinical trials, and the nonconventional therapies. But clearly understand this: Most alternative (nonconventional) approaches are altogether different from protocols being scientifically tested in authorized clinical trials. This makes them the choices of last resort. Make certain you have fully explored the conventional treatment options first. After all, this is what survivors do! Take a lesson from their success.

Allow yourself time to reflect on these important decisions. Don't be pressured by anyone to hurry a decision that would make you uncomfortable. When the treatment recommendations are consistent, and the people who administer the treatment have your confidence, and you can say with conviction that this is what you should be doing now, then, and only then, are you ready to go to the next step.

AN IMPORTANT THING YOU CAN DO

Take out your wellness notebook and thoughtfully, carefully, and systematically reflect on your treatment decision. Take another break. Reflect.

# #11

# DECIDE!

There is power in deciding. Without the power of a definite decision, all the analysis in the world will lead you nowhere.

The cancer journey is made up of little decisions and big decisions. Your treatment program is a big decision. In many ways this decision will determine the direction of your entire life. Now is the time to decide.

Decision is the spark that ignites action. Until a decision is reached, nothing happens.

Making decisions like this takes courage. But there is power in facing the fact that you have cancer, then carefully doing your homework, and finally deciding on a course of action. Without exercising your courage, the problem will remain forever unaddressed.

Decide! Do not straddle the fence or make a partial decision. This is the time to take a firm stand on one side or another, the time to *make a full commitment*.

Yes, you will monitor your decision. You will keep your options open, of course. But now is the moment to say, "This is how we will climb the mountain! Now let's get started!"

Decision frees us from many of the uncertainties caused by fear, doubt, and anxiety. Yes, there is risk. But there is greater risk in making no decision, hoping that all will magically be well.

Decide. You've done the work. This is not blind chance. This decision is the culmination of careful and sustained inquiry. Now is the time for action.

Decision awakens the spirit. Do you feel and sense that part of you springing to life? Nourish that spirit. Cherish it. It is the life force inside of you working for you, helping you get well again.

Decide. The decision comes first, the results follow. Today is the day. Now is the hour. This is the moment! Decide!

### AN IMPORTANT THING YOU CAN DO

Now, make the treatment decision. And feel the power of the spirit that deciding generates.

# #12

## GIVE
## ONLY
## *INFORMED*
## CONSENT

All treatment decisions should be made—must be made—with the informed consent of the patient or patient's guardian. This means you need to know in detail, in terms you can clearly understand, all the risks entailed in any surgery, anesthesia, or similar procedure.

You'll be asked to sign a consent form. *Do not sign a blank consent form.* Make certain that the exact procedure is described and that you fully understand it. You have the right to set limits on these documents. You can cross out statements you do not care to consent to. For example, I drew a line through the section of my consent form that asked my permission to videotape the operation for the removal of my lung.

You have the right to refuse treatment. An adult who is mentally competent can refuse treatment even if it may result in death. Nancy was a young woman who was pregnant. Even though she was advised to go ahead with treatment for lung cancer, she felt so strongly about the potential harm to her unborn child that she elected to postpone treatment until after her delivery. She exercised her right to refuse consent.

You need to understand clearly and completely what you are consenting to. Gary, a retired pilot who made his home in Oregon, recognized that something was wrong with his health when he began to feel weak all the time. During the last six months he had lost more than twenty pounds without dieting. "I just wasn't hungry," he said. "And I felt like I had a low-grade fever much of the time." Then Gary became aware of swelling in his abdomen.

Finally he went to his doctor, who ordered a variety of tests. There was a complete physical examination, the most thorough he had ever experienced. Then came chest X-rays, CAT scans, a blood work-up, urine tests, and more. After consulting with other specialists, the doctor finally told Gary he had Hodgkins disease.

Gary signed a consent form that said *laparotomy*, thinking that he was giving permission for a biopsy. "The way it was presented," said Gary, "this seemed like just another test to determine, with more certainty, the extent of the disease. The doctor told me they needed to know where the cancer had spread. I thought it was no big deal and that I'd be out of the hospital the next day."

In fact, a laparotomy is a surgical procedure that allows the doctors to explore the entire abdominal area. It is major surgery that should only be done by a team of experienced surgeons. Because of complications and infections, Gary's hospital stay lasted two and a half weeks. It left him with significant scars and lasting discomfort, while not confirming the spread of the disease.

While Gary technically gave consent to the procedure, in his mind he had given his okay for something much different. "I should have asked," lamented Gary. "But it seemed like a minor procedure."

Your doctor is obligated to inform you fully of any procedure you are being asked to consent to. This means explaining to you the procedure's purpose, risks, other alternatives, and the risk of *not* having the procedure. Don't be intimidated by the medical lingo. Make certain you get this information in language you understand. More important, make certain you ask detailed questions prior to giving any consent. Don't tolerate a physician's attitude that your concerns are unwelcome. If he or she is condescending or overly impatient, find another doctor. And be certain to include on your list of questions, "Why is this absolutely necessary?"

### AN IMPORTANT THING YOU CAN DO

Ask your physician, not an associate, an assistant, or a nurse, to describe clearly the risks involved in your tests and treatment. Compare the risks to the expected benefits.

# #13

# Believe
# in Your
# Treatment
# Program

*Excited belief.* This is one of the great intangibles in a successful treatment program. Excited belief is a natural extension of your conviction about your treatment decision. And it is your personal responsibility to believe in and be excited about your treatment program.

Rachael and May both attended one of the Cancer Conquerors Foundation's Cancer Survival Training Seminars in Atlanta. Rachael is a Georgia homemaker who started a course of radiation following surgery for breast cancer. Her attitude toward treatment was "I guess it's something I have to do."

May received virtually the same diagnosis about a month after Rachael's. May also had surgery and a follow-up course of chemotherapy. But her attitude was totally different from Rachael's: "I saw those chemicals as a great healing agent, something coming into my body to make me well. I welcomed my chemotherapy with open arms!"

Today May is free of cancer. Rachael continues to struggle.

Cancer survivors develop a confidence and an excited belief in their treatment programs that other patients simply do not possess. I am convinced that a correlation exists between belief in one's treatment and the effectiveness of that treatment program. This observation leads me to respect the awesome power of the mind and the human spirit in the cancer journey.

Colleen is a California wife, mother, and elementary school teacher. After three years of remission, she had a severe recurrence of breast cancer. The disease was now in her liver and bones. Her doctors gave her less than a year to live. "I knew I was at the crossroads," said Colleen. "And when I learned that survivors held an excited belief about their treatment, I decided I'd better do the same." Now, more than five years later, Colleen is cancer-free.

I realize that this is only anecdotal evidence and cannot stand up to scientific scrutiny. But I have seen beliefs and attitudes like May's and Colleen's make the difference in so many cases that to me the correlation between belief in treatment and effectiveness of treatment is fact.

I predict that someday the scientific and medical communities will document the biochemical reality of this kind of optimism. In the meantime, I suggest you not enter the debate. Instead, go with the survivors and develop an excited belief about your treatment.

### AN IMPORTANT THING YOU CAN DO

"Own" your treatment program. See it as a friend. Believe it is there to help you. Excited belief! That's what you are after.

# #14

## OVERCOME NAUSEA

One of the realities for about half of the cancer patients undergoing treatments is nausea and/or vomiting. Most people can significantly improve this situation, but it takes some experimentation. Here are some suggestions:

- Ask your oncologist for antinausea medication. There are now many alternatives and more coming on the market each day. Some are particularly effective when taken about thirty minutes before eating.
- Use relaxation exercises. (See #34)
- Eat smaller meals more often. Try six daily meals.
- Emphasize low-fat foods, especially fresh fruits.
- Limit liquids taken with meals. Drink no liquids the hour before meals and the hour following meals. But be sure to take in enough liquids at other times.
- Clear cool liquids are recommended. Iced herb teas, ginger ale, clear broths, popsicles, or apple-juice ice cubes are worth trying. Take all liquids slowly.

- Eat dry foods—crackers, toast, popcorn—especially at the start of the day or the first sign of nausea. Sorry, no butter on the popcorn.
- Eat salty foods. Avoid overly sweet foods.
- Do not lie down for two hours after eating. You can rest sitting up. Or if you simply must stretch out, prop a couple of pillows under your head to gain elevation.
- Sometimes loose clothing or fresh air will help in nausea control.

### AN IMPORTANT THING YOU CAN DO

Experiment with the above ideas. They have proven successful for many other cancer patients.

# #15

## Make the Most of Your Appointments

Free and open communication between you and your entire medical team is one of the most important facets of your cancer recovery journey. You need to stay informed. You want feedback. But seldom does this come voluntarily. You'll have to ask for it.

Smart patients bring a list of questions to virtually every medical appointment. If you have continuing or new symptoms, ask about them. If you are experiencing side effects, ask about them. Ask for further information about issues you have learned of from your reading or from talking to other patients.

"My radiation technician started to tease me about all my questions," said a retired Minneapolis professor who was being treated for prostate cancer. "I'd walk in the room and she'd say, 'What's on your list today Dr. Nelson?' But I was determined to participate fully, to be an active patient. So I didn't let her remarks bother me in the least."

Speak with total honesty to your doctor and the entire medical team. They are not mind readers. Tell them your problems and ask for their opinions. Bring a family member with you if you have trouble being assertive. He or she can be your wellness advocate. Many people are intimidated by their doctors. If you are one of these people, recognize it and act immediately to remove that needless hurdle. If you are having trouble understanding and absorbing medical information, bring a tape recorder. Then you'll be able to review explanations and instructions at your convenience.

In case this hasn't been emphasized enough by now, know that your ability to *ask questions* is one of your most significant powers. When in doubt, write down your questions and then read them from the list.

If you truly want to make the most of your medical appointments, get in the habit of expressing your sincere gratitude to your medical team. A group of doctors at a large county hospital in Pennsylvania lamented to me, "We try so earnestly to help a patient. I wish once in a while they would simply say, 'Thank you.'" I can remember giving an appreciative hug to my oncologist. From that day forward I was treated like royalty in that office. Start showing your appreciation to these very important people in your life. Remember, they're people who respond to you just as you respond to them.

### AN IMPORTANT THING YOU CAN DO

Use your wellness notebook to record both your questions and the answers you are given. Keep the notebook handy. Bring it to your appointments. If you rely on your memory, or record your questions on bits of paper scattered here and there, you'll never have timely and accurate information. And write a thank-you note to your medical team after your next visit.

# #16

## Monitor
## Your
## Progress

As you continue your treatment program, you'll be given tests to determine how well it's working. Ask about the tests prior to agreeing to them. Then insist that the doctor share the results.

It's a real uplift to know that you are making progress. But even receiving a response that is less encouraging than you hoped can have a positive side. It should lead you and your doctor to consider other forms of treatment. Many exist. If all standard therapies have been exhausted, perhaps now is the time to ask about investigative treatments.

It is your responsibility to monitor your treatment program. Don't wait. Ask.

### AN IMPORTANT THING YOU CAN DO

Ask your doctor how and when he or she will check the progress of your treatment program. Then be certain that it happens.

# CHAPTER FOUR

## HEAL
## YOUR
## LIFE-STYLE

Several years ago a Stanford health newsletter estimated that life-style issues such as diet, exercise, and general health habits accounted for 61 percent of the premature deaths due to cancer. The proportional contribution of genetics was 29 percent, and medical services themselves were listed as contributing to 10 percent of premature cancer deaths.* The point is obvious: Life-style is critical in the survival journey.

Life-style issues are a matter of personal choice. Clearly, there is much we can do to help ourselves get well again by making these choices. Let's examine how thousands of cancer survivors have helped in their own healing.

*Stanford Heart Disease Prevention Program Newsletter

# #17

---

# LIVE
# "WELL"

Wellness is a way of living, a life stance and a life-style that one can choose in order to achieve the greatest potential for total well-being.

Wellness is balance. Wellness encompasses body, mind, and spirit.

Wellness recognizes and acts on the fact that everything one thinks, says, does, feels, and believes has an impact on one's well-being.

Wellness can be chosen at any moment, in any circumstance, regardless of physical condition.

Conquering cancer demands that you reach beyond the physical issues of illness. Your mental, emotional, and spiritual health has a powerful effect on your well-being.

Kelly is a forty-eight-year-old account executive with a major investment firm. He developed malignant melanoma. "I went through the surgery and radiation just as recommended," said Kelly. "But I knew the real problem. I wasn't taking care of myself." Kelly hadn't exercised for years. His diet and nutrition habits were deplorable. He despised his work. And his marriage was coming apart.

Like so many survivors, Kelly considered cancer his "wake-up" call: "I realized my life was off-course in many ways. And I knew it was up to me to change it."

These are common sentiments expressed by many survivors of cancer. They see their illness as a message to make life changes, and they take personal responsibility for doing so. Kelly went on to say, "When I quit my job and opened a floral shop, my entire life started to heal. Cancer has actually been very good for me."

Exercising the decision to take personal responsibility for one's total well-being is very common among cancer survivors. This is whole-person wellness, a way of living the rest of your life no matter what the length.

This natural, total well-being does not have conditions attached to it. "Without conditions" means that although your wellness may be *obscured* by illness, it is a matter of personal choice whether your wellness will be *destroyed* by illness. It is possible to discover high-level wellness in the very midst of life-threatening illness.

The decision to live "well" is significant and profound. Never again will your well-being be a static state measured simply by the lack of physical symptoms, a place where you just get and stay well. Wellness becomes a quest to nurture one's emotional and spiritual well-being while honoring one's physical needs.

### AN IMPORTANT THING YOU CAN DO

Start the quest. Open your mind to whole-person wellness. In your wellness notebook, write down one step you can take today to improve your greater well-being. Then write down one step you can take today to eliminate something in your life that does not support your greater well-being. Now act, doing what is clearly do-able today. Determine to live life at a new level of wellness no matter what the length.

# #18

## OPERATE
## UNDER
## NEW
## ASSUMPTIONS

Compare the assumptions behind conventional health care versus whole-person wellness:

**ASSUMPTIONS BEHIND CONVENTIONAL HEALTH CARE:**

1. The patient is reliant upon the medical community.
2. The professional is the authority.
3. Symptoms are treated, not investigated.

4. Specialized and concerned with body's subsystems.
5. Body viewed as a series of mechanical functions.

**ASSUMPTIONS BEHIND WHOLE-PERSON WELLNESS:**

1. The patient has, or should develop, independence.
2. The professional is a healing partner.
3. The underlying causes are sought *and* the symptoms are treated.
4. Unified and concerned with person's whole life.
5. Body viewed as a changing system.

6. Primary repairs made with surgery or drugs.

6. Intervention is minimal and appropriate. Noninvasive therapies are used when possible.

7. Pain and illness are purely negative.

7. Pain and illness are messages to value and act on.

8. Mind and emotions are a secondary factor in health.

8. Mind and emotions are a major factor in health.

9. Body and mind are separate.

9. Body and mind form one unit and always affect each other.

10. Disease prevention is largely environmental; not smoking, attention to diet, exercise, and rest.

10. Wellness means prevention plus wholeness: harmony in relationships, work, goals; a balance of body, mind, and spirit.

There is an important issue behind these assumptions. Your medical team will be helpful in addressing just one part of your cancer journey, the physical disease portion. Wellness encompasses far more. Total whole-person wellness is our goal, and the responsibility for achieving it falls to each of us personally.

### AN IMPORTANT THING YOU CAN DO

Review the above assumptions. Circle those assumptions you believe. Are you a traditionalist? Or do you identify with the spirit of whole-person wellness? What does this tell you to do? How might you be best served?

# #19

## SCHEDULE YOUR WELLNESS

All important tasks demand a schedule. And there is no more important work in your life right now than the work of getting well again.

The trouble is, most people keep putting off the work of wellness, thinking they will get to it later. And guess what? They seldom, if ever, get around to it. Or if they do, it's only after everything else that is "important" has been taken care of.

Develop the attitude that there is nothing more important in your life right now than your work of wellness. For the time being, your wellness efforts need to take priority over family, job, community or religious activities, and social obligations. Getting well is your new top priority.

I actually blocked out my week on a schedule. Here's what a typical weekday looked like while I was in the middle of recovery:

| | |
|---|---|
| 6:00 A.M. | Wake up |
| 6:15 | Exercise |

| | |
|---|---|
| 6:45 | Meditate |
| 7:00 | Shower, eat, and commute |
| 9:00 | Work |
| Noon | Lunch and meditate |
| 1:00 P.M. | Work |
| 4:30 | Commute |
| 5:30 | Meditate |
| 6:00 | Dinner |
| 7:00 | Family time |
| 9:00 | Read and meditate |
| 10:00 | Sleep |

Doctors appointments were worked in as needed. During commutes I virtually always listened to wellness tapes. And weekends found me devoting even more time to study and meditation. Throughout the entire process, I became more gentle with myself, demanding less in the way of outside activities and more in the way of self-care. I took control of my schedule and made wellness my top priority.

### AN IMPORTANT THING YOU CAN DO

Start a new page in your wellness notebook. Make a schedule for your week similar to mine. Minimize obligations that cause undue stress. Give ample "core time" to the upcoming wellness disciplines discussed in this book.

---

I suggest you take a break from your wellness work after completing your schedule. Start the next section tomorrow or after you have rested. In the meantime, give careful consideration to how you spend your time. Modify your schedule to meet your new wellness priorities.

# #20

---

## STOP
## ALL
## USE
## OF TOBACCO

It totally mystifies me how some cancer patients can continue to smoke. John had colon cancer. After surgery he started a course of chemotherapy. But do you think he quit smoking? No! "I don't have lung cancer," he'd say as he smiled and left our Cancer Survival Training sessions.

If I could say this any more strongly I would. *If you are a user, cut out any and all tobacco immediately.* Cigarettes, cigars, chewing tobacco—all must go. There is no excuse, even nicotine addiction, that is sufficient to continue this harmful habit that is putting cancer-causing chemicals into your body.

The question is not whether you *can* quit. The question is whether you *will* quit. I know this firsthand. I started smoking when I was in my late teens. There is no doubt in my mind that smoking directly contributed to my lung cancer just over twenty years later. In those twenty years I seriously tried to quit five or six times. Willpower alone didn't get the job done. A change in thinking, a different self-perception did. I first went from perceiving myself as a smoker to seeing myself as a person who chose to smoke. I detached emotionally and psychologically from my cigarettes. Then, in my mind, I told my smoking behavior to leave my life because I now perceived myself as a nonsmoker. This can work for you too.

If you are not a smoker, great! Keep it up. But eliminate your exposure to secondhand smoke. Always sit in the nonsmoking sections of restaurants. Ask your smoking co-worker to have his or her cigarette outside. You can take charge of this condition too!

It has never been more important for you to strive for maximum health. Tobacco use, and even exposure to tobacco smoke, has no place in the quest for wellness.

### AN IMPORTANT THING YOU CAN DO

Stop all tobacco use immediately. Wean yourself with a nicotine patch if you need to. And stay away from tobacco users while they are smoking.

# #21

## ADOPT
## THIS
## DIETARY
## STRATEGY
## DURING
## TREATMENT

There has never been a more important time in your life to eat well than during your treatment for cancer. Recovery from cancer demands premium-grade fuel to succeed fully. Your dietary and nutritional habits can make a significant contribution to your getting well again. Here's the basic winning strategy:

1. *Maintain Weight*. Maintain a diet that is high enough in calories to keep up your normal healthy body weight. Weigh yourself each week and record the results in your notebook. This is no time to start a crash diet.

2. *Emphasize Protein*. Eat foods that are high in protein. The best sources are nonfat dairy foods, grains, legumes, seeds, and nuts. Your protein and calorie needs are greater during treatment and recovery than normal. Emphasizing protein will help keep your energy level high, maintain strength, and rebuild normal tissue affected by treatments.

3. *Raise Food Quality*. Eat premium foods, meaning those that are minimally processed. Look first for fresh fruits, fresh vegetables, and whole grains. If a food is boxed, bottled,

canned, or frozen, it has most often been processed and lacks the nutritional content of the fresh alternative.

## AN IMPORTANT THING YOU CAN DO

Determine that during treatment you will eat better than you have in your entire life. The strategy: maintain weight; eat plenty of protein; and choose premium foods.

# #22

---

## FOLLOW
## THESE
## "EAT SMART"
## GUIDELINES

Unless your physician has prescribed a special diet, there are some "eat smart" guidelines that you would be wise to follow in overcoming your cancer:

- When in doubt, eat a plant. Fresh fruits and fresh vegetables are now your foods of choice.
- Eat breads and pastas that are made from whole grains.
- Look to grains and legumes for protein. Try brown rice with any type of bean. Obtain additional protein by sprinkling chopped nuts over steamed vegetables and fresh salads. Limit chicken and turkey. Eliminate red meats. ("Flesh" foods are difficult to digest fully and have been linked by some researchers to stomach, bladder, liver, breast, and colon cancers.) If you must have animal protein, try water-packed tuna and steamed or broiled fish.
- Use low-fat or nonfat dairy products. Even some cheeses and ice creams are now made with low-fat or skim milk.

- Use monosaturated fats like canola, olive, and peanut oils whenever possible. If you have to fry, use a nonstick spray.
- Use fat- and sugar-reduced products whenever possible. Do your best to limit consumption of foods with fat and sugar substitutes.
- Consume caffeine and alcoholic beverages, and salt-cured, pickled, and smoked foods only in moderation.

### AN IMPORTANT THING YOU CAN DO

Keep a food diary in your wellness notebook during the next week. Write down everything you eat. Compare your diet with the above list. Is there any room for improvement?

# #23

## REPLACE
## FLUIDS

Are you looking for a simple action that will vastly increase your opportunity for survival and recovery? Here it is: Drink the equivalent of eight cups of water each and every day! Not coffee. Not soda. Water.

It is an almost universal truth—people with cancer are dehydrated. Lack of water inhibits the immune system, the most potent defense you have against cancer. The environment your cells live in is not blood, it is fluid. The lymph system, a key component of your immune system, is a fluid system requiring adequate water to function at its highest capacity.

Through natural elimination, perspiration, and even breathing, your body loses water daily. Fluid simply must be continually replaced in appropriate quantities for you to be optimally well.

I prefer water with no chlorine or fluorides. This is difficult to get from most municipal water systems. Even bottled water, especially if contained in plastic, is not a sure answer.

Some research indicates that sunlight starts a chemical reaction in the plastic bottle that can result in carcinogens in the water.

How can you get pure water? I recommend a water purification system in your home or certified chemical-free spring-fed bottled water in glass containers.

### AN IMPORTANT THING YOU CAN DO

Drink eight 8-ounce glasses of pure water each day.

# #24

## KNOW
## WHY
## YOU'RE
## EATING

Long-term dietary changes require more than shifts in our menus. Eating is so much a part of our lives that any permanent change must involve not only *what* we eat but also *why* we eat.

We sometimes allow our immediate frame of mind rather than our bodies to regulate our diet. A compulsion to satisfy our emotions, to handle our anger, frustration, worry, boredom, or guilt, is often easily accomplished by eating. When this happens we have become a slave to our emotions, something we can choose not to do.

Some people develop an attitude that changing their diet is something they *have to* do. I suggest you try an outlook that reflects the fact that a change in diet is contributing to getting well again—something you *get to* do!

If you want to eat with awareness, consider these proven tips:

- Don't keep any high-fat foods around the house where they will be a serious temptation.

- Make a rule of not eating in front of the television, where you don't pay attention to what or how much you eat.
- Don't eat so quickly that you can't enjoy your food. It takes about twenty minutes for our brains to realize that our stomachs are full. Slow down. Take a break midmeal.
- Reward appropriate eating behavior, but don't use food as the reward. If you've had a good week or have reached a wellness goal, treat yourself to a concert or a new outfit. (Don't punish yourself with guilt if it hasn't been a good week. Just don't reward yourself. Try again next week.)
- Make each meal a pleasant experience. Stop eating on the run or while standing at the kitchen counter. Take time to put out a place setting. Offer a short affirmation or prayer of gratitude for each meal. You'll then be nurturing yourself emotionally and spiritually, as well as physically, at every meal.

### AN IMPORTANT THING YOU CAN DO

Distinguish between a food craving, which is a psychological need, and hunger, which is the body's need for nourishment. Check your urge to eat the next time you see a food advertisement. A craving diminishes when we take on another activity. Go for a walk. Call a friend. Read a book. Then evaluate. Was it a craving or hunger? Honor your hunger, not your craving. Eat with awareness!

# #25

# DECIDE ON NUTRITIONAL SUPPLEMENTS

Even though most people in the medical community will not endorse the practice of nutritional supplementation, most cancer survivors believe in and use vitamin and mineral supplements. But it is absolutely essential to emphasize that survivors take these vitamins and minerals *in addition to, not in place of,* conventional medical therapy. Once I understood how widespread supplementation was among survivors, I decided to follow suit.

Each patient is responsible for his or her own decisions on this issue. The problem is, the whole field has an uncertain reputation, and as you explore it, you'll find people making incredible claims that just do not stand up to scrutiny. So be very careful, even skeptical.

I was helped by a nutritional therapist. And after much study and consultation, I adopted the following supplementation program:

| SUPPLEMENT: | DAILY DOSE: |
|---|---|
| Beta carotene | 25,000 iu |
| Vitamin C (powdered) | 10,000 mg |

| | |
|---|---|
| Vitamin E | 400 iu |
| Vitamin B complex | 50 mg |
| Folic Acid | 400 mcg |
| Pantothenic acid | 50 mg |
| Potassium | 500 mg |
| Selenium | 50 mcg |
| Zinc | 30 mg |

I stress that this was *my* approach. These are not specific recommendations for any individual. You must do your own research and design your own supplementation program. Or you may say "No thanks!" to the whole idea of nutritional supplements. The decision is up to you. I can only report that most survivors supplement.

### AN IMPORTANT THING YOU CAN DO

Telephone a professional nutritionist. Ask if he or she has experience in the therapeutic use of nutrition for cancer. If so, make an appointment for a consultation. And go to the library and your local bookstore. Start your own nutritional research today.

# #26

---

## MAKE EXERCISE PART OF YOUR RECOVERY PROGRAM

Hundreds of cancer survivors helped me make an important discovery: Exercise has a strong correlation with getting well. Virtually every person I interviewed talked about keeping physically active. Even people who were incapacitated or who needed a wheelchair emphasized their commitment to a regular exercise program.

Cancer survivors differed, however, in their exercise goals. Very few set out to run a marathon or become Olympic athletes. Instead, the most common exercise goal among cancer survivors was to experience an *increase in energy*.

I chose walking as my exercise. At first I was so weak that even a couple of minutes of walking was too much. So I began with simple arm circles—doing the backstroke movement with my arms fully extended. I'd do ten sets forward and follow with ten sets in the reverse direction. Soon I felt that increase in energy—the deeper breathing, the increase in heart rate, and the better skin color.

Amazingly, I began to feel stronger. Exercise really was

working! So I added the walking back into my exercise routine. Initially I would walk for perhaps five minutes before feeling an increase in energy. But soon that stretched to ten minutes. Over the months the exercise periods became longer. I bought an exercise book and added some full-body stretching routines before the start of my walk. And I ended the exercise session with some light calisthenics. I began to feel the combination of physical and emotional regeneration working together to enhance my overall well-being. You can experience the same thing.

Today I believe I have found the right balance. Hardly a day passes that I do not walk for at least thirty minutes. I precede the walk with about three minutes of full-body stretches and conclude the session with five minutes of push-ups and sit-ups.

This did not happen overnight. I determined this to be my correct level over a period of two years. Several times I have experimented with exercise beyond the normal thirty-five- to forty-minute daily routine. I tried walking for an hour each day but found I was experiencing hip soreness. I tried adding weight lifting only to realize I didn't enjoy it.

Some people think more exercise is better. "Why stop?" I've been asked. "If I feel good, shouldn't I just keep going?" I don't recommend it. Between the threat of injury associated with extended exercise and the rigid, grinding routine that often results in burnout, I believe more harm than good can come from workouts that last two or three hours daily.

Instead, find a type of exercise that you enjoy. Then pursue that routine just until you feel an increase in energy. That was the key for me. The physical benefits have included increased flexibility, strength, and cardiovascular capacity, weight loss, and lower blood pressure. But the psychological benefits are even greater. They have included joy, enthusiasm, and mental vitality. What a payoff!

Make exercise part of your cancer-recovery program. Believe it, exercise is for you! No matter how long it has been since you have exercised, no matter how incapacitated or confined you are, there are exercises you can do. And exercise will help you get well again.

### AN IMPORTANT THING YOU CAN DO

After an okay from your doctor, exercise just until you feel an increase in energy. This is your only exercise goal. Do the same tomorrow. Keep extending the duration as you build strength and stamina. No more excuses! Take charge. Your body will respond to your getting-well signals.

# #27

## GET
## MORE
## SLEEP

"I was always so tired. My radiation treatments drained me," noted Olivia, following her recovery from breast cancer. "I just wanted to sleep all the time. But with all my responsibilities, who had time to be sick or to sleep?"

Fatigue is part of nearly every cancer patient's journey. Unfortunately, many patients interpret fatigue as an indication of their quickly approaching demise. This is not necessarily so.

During and just after treatment, you are physically a different person. Just look at what is happening to you. With surgery, a major wound has been inflicted on your body. Chemotherapy puts chemicals into your system that change who you are on a biochemical level. Radiation causes cellular alterations in your body. Repairs demand rest. No wonder cancer patients are tired.

"For three months I cut back to half days on my work schedule," said Ted after his bout with bladder cancer. "I took an afternoon nap for a year following my treatment," said Alicia, who recovered from ovarian cancer. "I still take afternoon naps," said Bert, celebrating his six-year anniversary from a lung cancer diagnosis.

The fact is, *survivors rest.* It can be a major mistake to carry on at the same pace to which you were accustomed when you were totally healthy. Feeling tired is normal for anyone with any illness. During treatment you may feel tired for weeks until your body gets the opportunity to adjust and recover.

Provided you are getting adequate food and moderate exercise, fatigue is nothing to consume you with worry. It is not a sure sign of your demise. Practice deep relaxation as you start your meditations. Take that morning nap. Add an afternoon nap if you require it. Or a short rest before dinner may be just what is needed. And eight or more hours of sleep each night is an absolute essential.

### AN IMPORTANT THING YOU CAN DO

Give yourself permission to get more sleep. Block out rest times on your wellness schedule. Allow your body the rest it needs to heal.

# #28

# FIND A
# POSITIVE
# SUPPORT
# GROUP

You need a support group. It is no accident that cancer patients who regularly attend support-group meetings live longer than those who do not. In the late 1980s a research team at Stanford University confirmed what cancer survivors have known for decades. In a study of patients with advanced breast cancer, those who attended a weekly two-hour session had a life expectancy *twice* that of the nonattenders. We truly need one another for survival.

Distinguish between the two major types of support groups: informational and psychosocial. The informational groups instruct on a wide variety of issues. Subjects might include types of cancer treatments, common side effects, exercises following breast surgery, or how to live with an ostomy. The idea behind this type of support group is simply to pass along information.

More important are the psychosocial support groups. These organizations typically conduct supportive/expressive therapeutic programs that focus on the emotional, psychological, and spiritual aspects of cancer. Look for those groups that take a stance of hope without denying the reality of the illness. At meetings you should expect to express your own fears and frustrations freely and to allow others in the group to do the same. Learn from the responses of the group members who have overcome cancer.

One warning: The biggest problem with any type of support group is that instead of encouraging personal growth, many groups quickly turn into a "pity party." While there is significant value in allowing people to talk out their problems, the discerning group needs to judge when the talking is therapeutic and when it is rehearsing, and reinforcing, a problem.

When a group of us started Cancer Conquerors, committing to support one another in our wellness quests, we made a pact early on. Each meeting would include a lesson—somebody leading a discussion on a principle. The emphasis was to be on the application of ideas that would help us take control of and contribute to our own healing. One week the subject would be managing stress, the next week meditation. We included the doctor-patient relationship, managing treatment side effects, beliefs and attitudes, family and social relationships, managing fears, the spiritual journey, and other constructive subjects. It was the smartest move we ever made. We have never had a pity party.

AN IMPORTANT THING YOU CAN DO

Check with your hospital or the American Cancer Society. Find and attend several support groups. Judge for yourself: Are they actively working toward wellness or conducting a pity party? If you don't find what you are looking for, perhaps you need to consider starting a group in your home. Thousands of patients have done so, benefiting themselves and others. Contact Cancer Conquerors for start-up information. You'll find the address on page 143.

# CHAPTER FIVE

## HEAL
## WITH
## THE MIND

Fighting cancer is much more than simply excising a tumor,
treating a malignancy with radiation, or injecting chemotherapy
into a vein. Harnessing your inner resources, including the
mind, is a powerful factor in the quest for survival. And the ba-
sics are really quite simple. Let's continue our work.

# #29

# READ
# AND STUDY
# THESE
# BOOKS

Knowledge is power. Educate yourself! Get these books and start to study:

ANDERSON, GREG. *The Cancer Conqueror.* Word, 1988/ Andrews & McMeel, 1990. My thoughts, experience, and encouragement to readers on how to integrate body, mind, and spirit.

BENSON, HERBERT AND MIRIAM KLIPPER. *The Relaxation Response.* Avon, 1976. The source for relaxation and meditation concepts and techniques.

BORYSENKO, JOAN. *Minding the Body, Mending the Mind.* Addison Wesley, 1987. How to manage stress and uncertainty and find manageable solutions.

COUSINS, NORMAN. *Anatomy of an Illness as Perceived by the Patient.* W.W. Norton, 1979. A personal story of forming a healing partnership with doctors to combat serious illness by supplementing conventional medical care.

FIORE, NEIL. *The Road Back to Health: Coping with the Emotional Side of Cancer.* Bantam, 1984. A psychotherapist's personal experience with testicular cancer and his thoughts on the psychosocial aspect of illness.

KUSHNER, HAROLD. *When Bad Things Happen to Good People*. Avon, 1983. Getting over the questions of guilt, blame, and "Why me?"

LESHAN, LAWRENCE. *You Can Fight for Your Life*. M. Evans & Co., 1977. The emotional aspect of cancer.

MORRA, MARION, AND EVE POTTS. *Choices: Alternatives in Cancer Treatment*. Avon, 1987. Comprehensive questions and answers about cancer treatment. Excellent resource listings.

SIEGEL, BERNIE. *Love, Medicine and Miracles*. Harper & Row, 1986. Stories about self-healing from a former surgeon's observations of cancer patients and support-group work.

SIMONTON, O. CARL, STEPHANIE MATTHEWS-SIMONTON, AND JAMES CREIGHTON. *Getting Well Again*. Bantam, 1978. Guides cancer patients to participate in recovery through medical care, imagery, and psychotherapy.

AN IMPORTANT THING YOU CAN DO

Visit your local bookstore or library. Ask for guidance. Become an expert on your illness and your wellness.

# #30

## DISCOVER
## YOUR
## BELIEFS

Many survivors radically change their beliefs about cancer and about life. And many consider this to be the most fundamental aspect of healing with the mind. Attitudes have to do with one's *state of mind*, with one's mental habits. Beliefs are something different; now we are talking about *convictions*, the implications of certainty surrounding mental positions.

There are three widely held beliefs that work *against* overcoming cancer:

1. A diagnosis of cancer means my certain death.
2. The treatment program for solving my problems is drastic, is of questionable effectiveness, and involves many unpleasantries.
3. This situation "just happened" to me and therefore there is little I can do to control it.

All of these beliefs are untrue! The truth about these statements is:

1. Cancer, no matter how advanced, may or may not mean death.
2. Solutions do exist and, no matter how dramatic, have the potential to be effective. The difficulties in recovery are far outweighed by the benefits.
3. Most illnesses do not "just happen." On some level, cause and effect may be at work here. This knowledge can work for you in your recovery. Your response to a problem is more powerful than the problem itself. There is much you can do.

Do beliefs affect recovery? Absolutely! Beliefs and expectations constantly contribute to actual experience in all areas of life, including the experience of cancer. And our beliefs can be chosen. The trouble is, we seldom *consciously* choose them. Perhaps they have been imposed upon us for many years, like the conventional wisdom surrounding cancer. Perhaps we've assumed beliefs from parents, co-workers, or friends. We have picked up other people's beliefs and made them our own. They may or may not be true or helpful. But they have mighty power.

What beliefs have you chosen? *Awareness* of our fundamental beliefs is often the first and certainly one of the most dramatic ways to improve our situations. If you are harboring the belief that cancer means death, challenge it! The fact is, there are long-term survivors of every type of cancer, even those patients who had been told by doctors that there was no hope. What about you?

AN IMPORTANT THING YOU CAN DO

Analyze your beliefs. In your wellness notebook, quickly complete the following sentences with the first thoughts/feelings that come to mind:

1. When I think of my cancer diagnosis, I think _____
_____.

2. I believe my cancer treatment is_____

_____.

3. The one thing I believe would best help me is_____

_____.


Analyze how your beliefs align with the truth. Talk to others—those who have successfully walked the cancer path. Discover what they believe. Choose to change your self-limiting beliefs today.

# #31

## "REFRAME" YOUR CANCER

Most cancer patients look upon their illness as the most overwhelming threat to their lives they've ever encountered. "I thought of cancer as a powerful evil force here to inflict great injury upon me," said Raymond, a retired restaurant owner who was battling cancer of the larynx. "It was the ultimate threat."

Raymond's words described his mental outlook. He saw cancer as a powerful evil force inflicting great injury, and the ultimate threat. It took weeks of counseling, but Raymond was finally able to view his cancer not as a threat but as a challenge. Cancer became something that stimulated him to look at his entire life. He ultimately made changes in his vocation, exercise routine, diet, and spiritual life. Cancer became Raymond's wake-up call. This is what it means to reframe the illness.

José's diagnosis of prostate cancer was the most frightening and unwelcome event in his fifty-eight years. Even though tests confirmed that the cancer had been discovered early and the prognosis was very good, his constant panicked thought process focused on his imminent demise. "I didn't just have cancer, I *was* cancer," said José.

Frank also had prostate cancer, but his was significantly more advanced than José's, with bone involvement. Through some of the most challenging of treatments, Frank made a commitment to honor his true needs. Unlike José, Frank made the critical distinction that he had cancer, the cancer did not have him. "I realized that my mind and spirit had cancer only if *I* allowed it," said Frank.

Frank's response demonstrates the power we have over cancer and our lives. It is not the circumstances of illness that we control so much as our reaction to them. Our reaction can make all the difference. When we reframe cancer, we respond differently. We acknowledge and nourish our inner strength, even in the face of doubt and fear. The threat subsides. We take on the challenge.

Fortunately, both stories have very happy endings. José was able to embrace Frank's belief. Today both men are doing well.

### AN IMPORTANT THING YOU CAN DO

Reframe cancer by nurturing three responses:

1. Cancer is not so much a threat as it is a challenge.
2. My experience of the illness will be largely determined by the way I think.
3. The way I think is something I can choose. I choose wellness.

# #32

## EVALUATE
## YOUR
## SELF-TALK

From the moment we awaken in the morning until we drift off to sleep at night, we experience a constant stream of mental chatter. When we have cancer, that self-talk is nearly all negative, filled with fears. It makes for a frightening life experience.

Marion called Cancer Conquerors in a state of panic, her mind reeling out of control. After the first couple of minutes, I began to jot down the first words of her sentences. Imagine her state of mind:

"The cancer is spreading ..." "I think my insurance is going to be canceled ..." "How am I going to pay for this?" "It's all such a burden ..." "I'm afraid of chemotherapy ..." "My husband can't deal with this ..." "I feel so frightened ..." "Why did this happen to me?" "There's nothing I can do."

There *is* something Marion can do! And you can, too. Believe it or not, we absolutely do choose our every thought. We may think the same thought over and over out of habit, but we are still responsible for that original choice. Analyze the thoughts you have been holding about cancer. That self-talk is the ancestor of your experience of illness and of life.

Lou is a woman who has every excuse needed to lead a life of despair. Childhood abuse, a turbulent early marriage, children in trouble, a toxic divorce, a child who ran away, a second husband who died in a work accident, a severe auto accident after which she was disabled for eight months, and then lymphoma. "My mind," explained Lou, "was always filled with thoughts of life being unfair and difficult, a battle to be fought."

Then Lou discovered this great truth: Thoughts are the ancestors of every life experience. And Lou made a massive change. She became aware that her troubles were all in her past, over and done with. What became important was what she was choosing to think and say and believe in this moment. The thoughts and words she chose right then were the ones creating her future. That was eight years ago. And today Lou is a healthy, whole, happy person.

### AN IMPORTANT THING YOU CAN DO

Notice what you are thinking at this moment. Is your self-talk negative or positive? Do you want your future to be an extension of these thoughts?

# #33

## CHOOSE
## A DAILY
## AFFIRMATION

Affirmations are statements of fact that are positive. They take the place of the negative mental chatter that may be gripping you. Affirmations serve to "make firm" the positive things about you and your circumstances. They are *consciously chosen* self-talk.

Put affirmations in the present. The phrase "I am grateful for life today" is much preferred over a future-tense alternative like "I will show gratitude for my life."

Your words are constantly doing one of two things: building you up or tearing you down, healing or destroying. So assert positively. You are not so much changing the situation as you are changing your thinking about the situation. And changing your thinking about the disease of cancer may be at the heart of experiencing wellness.

## AN IMPORTANT THING YOU CAN DO

Start now to use the affirmation "I am a picture of wellness."
    Or use some of these:

"I am now receiving unlimited wellness."
"Complete wellness is now mine."
"I enjoy life now, this is my moment."
"I am grateful for today!"
"As I sow wellness, I reap wellness."
"I am a 'carrier' of wellness."
"There is nothing in all the world I fear."
"My body is producing miracles."
"I am free from worry. I know peace."
"Wellness is mine, now."

# 34

# Manage
# Your
# Toxic
# Stress

Mismanaged stress only adds to the physical and mental anguish cancer brings. Stress works at cross-purposes to wellness, putting the mind in a state of confusion, blurring the focus needed for healing. But there is something you can do about stress. It's called the *relaxation response*. First named and described by Herbert Benson, M.D., (see section #29) a cardiologist and associate professor of medicine at Harvard Medical School, the relaxation response is a simple, effective, self-healing meditation technique for reducing the detrimental effects of all kinds of stress that we live with every day, particularly the stress associated with a cancer diagnosis.

Benson found that the relaxation response is even more effective when one chooses a focus word or phrase that is closely tied to one's spiritual beliefs. The idea is to pick a word or short passage that has meaning to you: a Christian might use "The Lord Is My Shepherd" from the Twenty-third Psalm; a Jewish person might choose  a nonreligious person might like the word "peace."

Pick a phrase with significant personal meaning. Dr. Benson calls this the *faith factor* and explains that it can greatly contribute to helping our minds manage stress more effectively.

The quest for daily self-renewal starts with a decision to handle our problems with a sense of equanimity. Eliciting the relaxation response, especially when coupled with the faith factor, can get our minds working for rather than against our wellness.

### AN IMPORTANT THING YOU CAN DO

Triggering the relaxation response is simple. Try these steps:

1. Find a quiet place, free from distractions, and sit in a comfortable position.
2. Pick a focus word or short phrase that is deeply rooted in your spiritual beliefs.
3. Close your eyes and relax your muscles, from toe to head, particularly relaxing the shoulder and neck area, where a great deal of tension is carried.
4. Breathe slowly and naturally. Repeat your focus word as you exhale.
5. Assume a passive attitude. When a distracting thought comes to mind, simply dismiss it and return to your focus word.
6. Practice this response for ten to twenty minutes twice a day.

# #35

---

## PRACTICE
## VISUALIZATION

An extension of the relaxation process is visualization, also called imagery. This is a valuable tool for helping you believe in your ability to recover from cancer. It is an extension of the relaxation response in that it is typically added at the end of the relaxation exercises.

The essence of visualization is to create mental pictures of your immune system and treatment effectively fighting the cancer; the cancer disappearing; and your body returning to health. Don't make visualization any more complicated than this.

Picture the cancer in either realistic or symbolic terms. For those who require a realistic image, you may want to consult a medical text to search out pictures of actual cancer cells. Most patients, however, use symbols. I've had people describe their cancer as sand, a lump of clay, even ice cubes. I saw mine as jelly. The most important criterion for picturing the disease is to think of the cancer as weak and confused. Don't give it power. Your imagery need not be literally correct. Its importance lies in the meaning you give the cancer. Whether you choose a realistic or symbolic image, make the cancer weak.

If you are receiving treatment, imagine it as strong and powerful, damaging the weak cancer cells while the healthy cells remain intact. And picture your immune system fighting the cancer and flushing it out of your body. Picture the cancer shrinking until it is all gone. If you are experiencing pain, picture your white blood cells flowing to that area and soothing the pain. Whatever the problem, give your body the command to heal itself, visualizing the process in a way that makes sense to you. End the imagery by seeing yourself well, free of disease, and filled with energy.

How has this benefited you? Most people's fears tend to decrease as the imagery process gives them a greater sense of control. Many researchers believe the mental process has a direct biochemical influence on the body, producing a physical response to a renewed sense of hope. The resulting changes in hormonal balance can eliminate immune suppressors, thus allowing the body maximum opportunity to heal.

Some people consider visualization to be a form of self-deception. "After all," they reason, "I know the tumor has been growing." Separate what is happening from what you want the outcome to be. It is possible, and beneficial, to picture the cancer shrinking even though it may, at this moment, be growing. This is not self-deception. It is self-direction and is necessary to beginning the pursuit of any life goal. At first, reality will lag behind the vision we have of the desired outcome. But that *vision* will tend to pull us in the direction we need to go.

How can you make this technique work for you? After evoking the relaxation response, try this:

1. Picture your cancer cells as weak and confused.
2. Create a mental image of your treatment and your immune system overcoming the cancer.
3. See your body's natural processes eliminating the disease from your system.

4. See the cancer shrink until it is gone.
5. Imagine yourself well and filled with zest for living.

### AN IMPORTANT THING YOU CAN DO

Evoke the relaxation response and follow it with a visualization exercise. Do this twice a day.

# #36

## MINIMIZE
## TREATMENT
## SIDE
## EFFECTS

Conventional wisdom holds that cancer treatments are ineffective and have drastic side effects. Don't believe it.

Treatments are becoming more effective every day. And new antinausea drugs are rapidly lessening the negative side effects that many cancer patients experience. Conventional wisdom needs to be challenged.

Equally important is the mind's role in the treatment program. In a clinical trial of a new form of chemotherapy, part of the group was given saline solution, sterile salt water. Fully 30 percent of this group lost their hair! It is common for patients to get nauseous, not during or after treatment but on their way *to* treatment. Add to this the legions of examples in which the same treatment results in radically different side effects for different patients, and what do you get? *The mind at work*. Beliefs turned into biological realities.

As patients, you and I may perceive treatments entirely differently. During one of our Cancer Survival Training seminars, I asked Carol, a woman with breast cancer, to draw a picture illustrating her chemotherapy. A few minutes later she returned with a drawing of a devil giving her poison. At that same seminar Rhoda told us that she had refused both chemotherapy and radiation because she saw them as toxic chemicals that were more threatening than cancer itself. When I asked Rhoda to draw pictures of both chemotherapy and radiation therapy, she returned with drawings of acid that had eaten through a tabletop and a beam of light that had blinded a baby in a stroller.

These negative perceptions of treatment stand in the way of the body's ability to respond favorably. Whenever a patient sees treatment as a friend, the positive perception starts to work favorably with the treatment. The best way to make treatment a friend is to make certain you "own" the treatment program, knowing that this is what *you* consider to be the very best alternative at this time.

You can program yourself for the most positive outcome possible by using a type of visualization that athletes have successfully employed in training. After evoking the relaxation response, picture yourself sitting in a chair or lying on a table having your treatment administered. In your mind's eye, see the cancer shrinking. Feel your strength returning. At the end of your imaginary treatment, you feel good and ready to enjoy all the gifts of your renewed health and greater well-being.

If you do this perhaps one hundred times prior to starting treatment, or even in the middle of a course of treatment, your body will respond with maximum capacity and minimal side effects to the actual treatment. Like an Olympic athlete, you will be living the event in your mind first. The body will get the message as to how it should respond in the real situation.

## AN IMPORTANT THING YOU CAN DO

View your treatment as a friend who is there to help you. Take time to "image" your treatment dramatically helping you. Envision yourself as well, free of any treatment side effects, and returning to radiant health.

The steps in this section are basic mind/body principles. There's much more to healing with the mind. You may want to continue your training with more reading, seminars, and perhaps personalized instruction. Start with the source list, #29.

# Chapter Six

## Wellness:
## Your
## New
## Life
## Perspective

It is difficult to imagine any benefit coming from the experience of cancer. With the frightening diagnosis, the myriad of treatment decisions, and the need to manage the treatment side effects, how could your cancer experience ever be used for good?

Yet thousands of survivors tell of the real and lasting changes in outlook and character that come directly from their cancer journey. A whole new life opens as a result of cancer. This is possible for you too.

# #37

---

## UNDERSTAND
## THE MESSAGE
## OF ILLNESS

When you "reframed" cancer, you began to see illness as more of a challenge than a threat. Now it is time to take this one step further. If cancer can be viewed as a challenge, what is the challenge about?

In my opinion, the challenge in illness is a message, a call, an opportunity, for personal growth. And in this part of the cancer journey lies the seed of true healing and lasting wellness.

Could cancer be a message signaling you to make changes in your life? We've already suggested some changes on the physical level—diet, exercise, all the life-style issues. Might there be more?

Many survivors view cancer as a call for personal transformation, not only of health habits but also of attitudes and self-image. The wise patient uses the experience of cancer as a turning point, a time to replace ineffective and limited ways of coping with life by substituting healthier, more effective methods of handling relationships, vocations, and social challenges.

I believe that all of us have a personal responsibility to respond to cancer in this manner. Such a response is in our power. However, as soon as I take this position, people cry, "On some level, you're suggesting I gave myself cancer!" Not so! We may have participated, but we did not purposely set out to give ourselves a serious illness. Don't read blame or guilt into the message of illness. Instead, understand that if we have participated in our illness, then by definition, we can participate in our wellness. That participation is centered around living life differently.

Patients who go through this process of "wellness work," seeking the message of illness, often discover a link between their physical, emotional, and even spiritual states and the onset of their illness. More important, an encouraging number of the survivors whom I interviewed could trace the beginning of their healing to their decision to change beliefs and behaviors. They were able to examine the message in illness and choose a response that changed their lives. You can, too. Ask yourself:

- *What high-stress events or changes happened in the year or two prior to diagnosis?* Death of a spouse or child, loss of a job, and financial setbacks are obvious candidates. Also include internal stresses, such as disappointment, major adjustments, or ongoing conflict in important personal relationships. Most survivors can identify several stresses in their lives prior to the onset of cancer.

- *What was my emotional response to these circumstances?* This is a measure of your participation. Don't read blame here. Participation simply means how you responded to the circumstances that may have caused stress. Might you have put others' needs before your own? Were there alternative ways of reacting? Did you give yourself permission to mourn a loss or did you determine not to show your emotions? Did you permit yourself to seek support during these stresses? How effective was your emotional self-care? Most survivors gain significant insight from a close examination of these questions.

■ *How might my reactions to stressful circumstances be changed?*
Could these circumstances and people be removed from your
life? If not, how can you balance them, honoring your own
emotional needs first? Have you even considered what your
true needs are? Have you truly attempted to find ways to meet
them, regardless of what you feel others may say or think?

AN IMPORTANT THING YOU CAN DO

Take a thorough and unflinching personal inventory. In your
wellness notebook, complete this exercise:

1. High-stress event(s) that occurred in the year or two prior to
diagnosis or recurrence included_____

_____

2. My three major emotional responses to these high stress
events were (a)_____
(b)_____(c)_____
3. I could have changed these circumstances by_____

_____

4. I could have changed my emotional response by_____

_____

Complete the inventory and then consider stopping your
wellness work for today. Carefully contemplate the important issues raised in this exercise.

# #38

## LIVE
## THIS
## MOMENT

Many people with a diagnosis of cancer needlessly pollute their lives by living in the past or in the future. Instead, their goal should be to live well with the time they do have, this very precious present moment.

How many times have you heard yourself say, "If only I hadn't done such and such"? "If only I hadn't smoked." "If only I'd taken better care of myself." "If only . . ." If only . . ." "If only . . ." We mire ourselves in the regrets of the past and miss the moment we have been given.

At other times we get caught in the fear of the future: "What if such and such happens?" "What if the cancer spreads?" "What if the chemo fails?" "What if . . ." "What if . . ." "What if . . ." Here we miss the present moment because we are consumed with what may happen in the future.

The answer: *present-moment living*. Live now. Live today. Live this hour. Live this minute to its very fullest. All of our regrets about the past, no matter how sincere, won't change history. And our worries about the future won't add even another minute to our lives. On the contrary, both fears and worries diminish our current minutes by detracting from their quality.

Are wellness and happiness completely dependent on bodily condition? I think not! Enjoy each moment. Appreciate the fact that even with cancer, you have life, here, now. Living each moment fully is the secret to wellness. It has nothing to do with the *quantity* of time we may be given. It has everything to do with the *quality* of this time. Don't put off living a full life until you are "better." *Start now!*

"I was consumed with worry," said Brenda, a non-Hodgkin's lymphoma patient, "not just over my cancer but . . . about my entire life. My parents were divorced and I worried about my mother. My dad traveled a lot and I worried about his airplanes crashing. What about my student loans that still hung over my head, unpaid for several years? Why couldn't I maintain a relationship with a man? Was I just an intractable failure at life? And then my illness, on top of it all."

Corwin was diagnosed with colon cancer at the age of fifty-six. "It [the cancer diagnosis] came two years after my business failed. All I could think of in those two years was what I should have done differently. If only I had not put so much emphasis on the new product line. Why didn't I see the downturn in the economy? Why did I extend so much credit to our number-one customer? I should have announced shorter work weeks or lay-offs much sooner. Why didn't I listen to the banker? How am I ever going to get out of debt? If only the family didn't have to suffer. Life is so unfair. I'm ruined."

Brenda and Corwin have a similar problem. Both are contaminating their present moments. Brenda's worries about the future assure her of little peace this minute. Corwin's life is consumed by thoughts of self-judgment that imprison him in the past. Neither is living in the moment. Yet their only chance to capture true wellness is found in the now. What is required is a shift in thinking from what Corwin might have done in the past or what may happen to Brenda in the future, to what they can do right here, right now.

*Our capacity for wellness is equal to our ability to understand that the past does not equal the future.* Living in the now frees us from an internal bondage that keeps us from following the wellness path.

The past is over. It cannot touch you unless you allow it to remain in your life. The future cannot harm you unless you create the future from your thoughts of fear. The only time that contains the power to change our lives is the present moment. Past, present, and future are not necessarily continuous. Just because you have cancer now does not predict with certainty that you will have it next year. You have power in this moment that can change your life. Exercise that power now!

### AN IMPORTANT THING YOU CAN DO

Relinquish any thoughts or judgments that hold you to the past. Give up any fears that keep you from creating a healthy future. Pick one activity this day, this moment, that brings you pleasure, contentment, and happiness. Do it now! Know that the supply of these moments is limitless, there for the taking, if you will only choose to do so. Here, in the present moment, find your wellness.

# 39

# TAKE
# TIME
# TO PLAY

How much time have you allowed yourself to *play* in the last week? If you answered "No time," you are a member of a large club. That's unfortunate.

Some people react negatively to the idea that we humans need to play. Many believe that "grown-ups don't play." Somehow we think that playing is not the mature thing to do. Challenge this thinking. Play is part of the work of wellness.

The need to honor our playful nature is very strong. Most of us just repress it. We would do well to give ourselves permission to play, actually scheduling play time in our daily calendars. We must then treat that time carefully, assigning it the same importance and priority as other areas of life, such as work and family.

Sometimes we get fooled into thinking we are playing when we really are not. Ed, who was diagnosed with bone cancer, was also a member of a barbershop quartet. He thought his singing was play. Then Ed began to look at his "play" more closely. He soon realized his singing wasn't play so much as it was competition, a pressure to win contests—a pressure he did not need. Ed dropped out of the quartet and substituted kite making, in which the competition was strictly self-imposed. What a valuable lesson!

Notice that you're never too tired to play. In fact, if you think you're tired, perhaps that is a signal that you *need* to play. Play builds energy reserves. It is a great contributor to wellness.

Here's a list of ten noncompetitive play activities:

1. Go to the beach.
2. Fly a kite.
3. Shoot baskets.
4. Ride a bike.
5. Draw a picture.
6. Write a poem.
7. Skip around the yard.
8. Sing.
9. Listen to music.
10. Take the scenic route.

### AN IMPORTANT THING YOU CAN DO

Make your own play list. Record it in your wellness notebook. Put down this book right now and go play for thirty minutes. Go! Do it!

# #40

## LAUGH
## FOR HEALING
## POWER

Norman Cousins made many contributions to our understanding of the power of our emotional and spiritual choices. But none is so vividly remembered as his emphasis on laughter. In his 1981 book *Anatomy of an Illness*, Cousins called laughter *internal jogging*. And since that time, science has confirmed that even something as simple as a laugh or a smile has a positive biochemical counterpart.

Lighten up! It will directly help your wellness. Just notice how relaxed you feel after laughing at a good story or watching a funny movie. It's wonderful!

Jack is an East Coast investment banking executive, successful, wealthy, the owner of a beautiful home in Westchester County, and the recipient of a metastatic prostate cancer diagnosis. "I thought, my God, I'm going to die. Cancer was the most serious threat I had ever faced," said Jack. Jack had radiation treatment at a Manhattan hospital where he met Delmar, an older man filled with stories and laughter and joy. Delmar had successfully completed the same treatment for prostate cancer some seven years ago. Now he volunteered three days a week at the hospital. "My job," said Delmar, "is court jester!"

For most of us seriousness is seen as a high virtue. We tend to think that a laugh or a giggle is childish behavior and certainly not appropriate for adults. Jack used to subscribe to this thinking, "After all," he remarked, "investment banking is serious business. And you have to be serious to be taken seriously."

Baloney! There is nothing inconsistent with being an adult and including laughter in your life. There is nothing wrong with being ill and pursuing a lighthearted approach to wellness. This need not be some demented form of denial. Instead, it can be the opportunity to let the hidden child in you come out once in a while. Get in touch with that exuberant, life-filled child. Enjoy playing with your own children or grandchildren. Laugh at yourself and your seriousness.

Jack continued, "Delmar taught me about living. When I stopped being so damned serious, I started to get well."

### AN IMPORTANT THING YOU CAN DO

Go ahead. Rent that comedy video. Watch your favorite sit-com. Go to the local comedy club or a silly movie. Laugh! Let those positive chemicals and hormones loose. It's healing.

# #41

## Evaluate
## Your
## Relationships

Other people. A husband or wife, a friend or a lover, child or relative, boss, co-worker, or employee—the list is endless. At times, all of life seems to be made up of relationships. How we get along with the significant people in our lives seems to determine, to a large extent, the quality of life we have. And the absence of relationships can also cause much disharmony and dissatisfaction. Like it or not, relationships are central to our experience of life and even our experience of illness.

Cancer survivors give time and energy to relationships that build them up. Survivors put "on hold" relationships that tear them down. Patricia shared in a support group meeting what this meant to her: "I had to move out. It was difficult, particularly leaving my two children. But I knew that was what I needed at that time. And I stayed away for nearly three months."

Patricia had married while in college and was expecting her first child before her husband had graduated from business school. Patricia put her educational goals behind those of her husband and never got her degree, something her husband seemed to hold over her.

"He was always criticizing me," Patricia said. "And I would yell back, trying to defend myself from attack. I'd bring up times when he disappointed me. And he would counter with a litany of my shortcomings. God, it became a vicious circle. So I got the hell out of there."

Was a marriage gone askew partly responsible for Patricia's cervical cancer? I believe so—and Patricia came to believe this as well. On some level, the breach in her marriage was linked to her physical problems. After establishing her medical-treatment program, she began to look at her relationship with her husband.

Credit Patricia with wanting her marriage to work. With the help of a marriage counselor she was able to better understand her part in the ongoing battles. The counselor helped Patricia recognize her choice of responses and also helped her select other appropriate reactions to her husband's remarks. Today the two of them are working on improving their relationship, and Patricia is cancer-free.

Our relationships with others often reflect the relationship we have with ourselves. Do you experience conflict with a coworker? Look within to understand the inner conflict you may carry. Does a child seem self-willed and impossible? Look within. Do you carry a belief that kids in general are willful and impossible?

This internal search is our only real point of influence. When we evaluate relationships, the central task is to look within, discovering the truth: The only way to change others is to change ourselves first.

Do healed relationships always equate with healed bodies? I think the two go together, but I can cite only anecdotal evidence. When we stop punishing ourselves and others for things that happened in the past, we are then free to move on to the work of total wellness. This often results in vast and rapid physical improvement.

Survivors evaluate their relationships. They change what they can, which is themselves, and make peace with the rest. This shift often results in a new level of wellness.

### AN IMPORTANT THING YOU CAN DO

Take an inventory of the ten most important relationships in your life. Number a page in your wellness notebook from one through ten and write the people's names down. Did you realize these were the ten most important people in your life? Are there any relationships that need to be put "on hold"? Indicate them. Are there any that need improvement? What is one thing you could change that would improve each of those relationships? Do you appreciate how important this work is to the achievement of wellness?

# #42

## GET
## BEYOND
## "WHY?"

It's the inevitable question cancer patients ask: "Why did this happen to me?"

The trouble with the "why" question is that we seldom like the answers we are given. We fight them, not wanting to accept. Some think cancer is a life-style issue: "He smoked." That may be true for some but does not stand up to scrutiny for all cancer patients or all smokers. Others say the "why" is environmental: "We've polluted the planet. We're all getting sick." That may explain some cases, but why is it that other people exposed to the same carcinogens remain perfectly healthy?

Religion tries to answer the "Why me?" question. I've been told by well-meaning people that God was using cancer to punish sin, to prevent sin, to correct the patient for his or her eternal profit, to draw unbelievers to God, and to help the patient and family members learn submission. Incredible!

Underneath "why" is blame. "Why" is another way of saying we are helpless and the situation is beyond our control.

Some people blame others, some blame circumstances, some blame parents, some blame doctors, some blame the environment, and some blame God. Affixing blame does not help. Affixing blame only creates helpless victims, something I trust by now you feel you are not.

The road to personal wellness starts when we stop asking "why" and begin to consider the question "Toward what end?" Another way of saying this is "For what purpose?" Or, "How can this be used for good?" Given that we have cancer, the best question to pose is "How can I make this experience benefit myself, others, and the world?"

## AN IMPORTANT THING YOU CAN DO

In your wellness notebook, start a new page with the heading *How I can make my experience of cancer beneficial.* Describe, in writing, how you believe cancer can help you and others physically, emotionally, and spiritually. Continue to add to this list as you travel your cancer journey and gain deeper insights.

# #43

## PRACTICE
## SELF-DISCIPLINE

Living the well life requires living with values and actions that may not be the easiest or most convenient to practice. On a rainy day it might be easier to stay in bed and forget the exercise. And instead of preparing a high-nutrition lunch, it might seem simpler to use the drive-through window of the nearest fast-food restaurant. Our *intention* to move toward wellness may seem strong. But too often our practices become weak.

Wellness self-discipline includes thought and deed, intent and practice. This principle is just as valid whether you are facing a just-baked batch of chocolate-chip cookies, a dark cold morning for exercise, or an "unforgivable" person. Gentle, wholesome self-discipline is at the core of making wellness real in your life. The issue is not whether we *can* choose wellness. It's whether we *will* choose wellness.

The practice of self-discipline leads to two very powerful life qualities: self-respect and freedom. When your walk matches your talk, when intent and action are one, you have a consistency in your life that is unshakable. You are grounded in a principle-oriented life experience, firm in the knowledge that what you are doing physically, emotionally, and spiritually is in your highest and best interest. Tremendous self-respect flows from that position. And when you are doing what is important to you, this leads to personal freedom, freedom from the traps of obsession, compulsion, and self-pity. This is personal power at the highest level, a strong and quiet inner assurance that is one of the best rewards of the wellness journey.

Wellness becomes a way of living, a disciplined way of life that is filled with self-respect. When I get up in the morning, the first thing I do is pull on my sweats and running shoes. No excuses. I discipline myself to exercise.

Diet was a wellness discipline that challenged me. I loved sweets, especially pastries. Today, I simply do not allow myself to indulge. Discipline.

Meditation—when did I have time to fit this into a busy schedule? Yet I do, twice each day. Discipline. Meditation gives a perspective on the balance of the day that I *will not* live without.

The same goes for a conscious purpose/play balance, nurturing my relationships, and honoring my spiritual needs. Each important area of my life requires that consistent disciplined practice in order for it to work to its potential.

"But you're in bondage to your disciplines," protested Manuel, a big burly mechanical engineer with kidney cancer who attended one of our workshops in San Antonio. "You're right," I responded, "and so are you." The issue is not bondage. The issue is which habits will we choose in our lives. I decided to discipline myself to choose the habits of wellness. The result is self-respect and freedom.

## AN IMPORTANT THING YOU CAN DO

Match your walk with your talk, your actions with your best intentions. Pick one area—perhaps diet or exercise—and make that your focus today. Then make it your focus for the next day, and the next, and the next . . . Feel your self-respect. Bask in the personal power and freedom this discipline gives you.

# CHAPTER SEVEN

## FOR
## THE COMMITTED

If you've been following and implementing the steps in this book, you're well on your way to a positive response to cancer. Many cancer survivors go even further, reaching higher levels of wellness in all areas of their lives. "Today, I am actually able to say cancer was the best thing that ever happened to me," claimed Donna, after a near-fatal recurrence of breast cancer. "My health, my life, has never been better!" This can happen for you, too.

# #44

---

## SEE
## LIFE
## THROUGH
## SPIRITUAL
## EYES

What do you *see* when you look at your life? Do you see a body riddled with disease, dreams hopelessly derailed, a family frightened and in despair?

Or can you see a precious moment, a special instant in space and time where mind and spirit are ill only if you allow it? Can you see the beauty and grace, even the perfection, in your life without coloring those qualities with the pain of cancer?

Peter was a forty-year-old father who developed pancreatic cancer. It was a difficult battle for Peter, especially since he wanted to live so very much. His valiant efforts were an inspiration to many. During one of our lengthy telephone sessions, Peter remarked, "I think the spiritual part began to make sense last night. We were at the dinner table, the whole family. And I saw something different. It has really stuck with me."

"What do you mean?" I asked.

"Well, before last night, I always saw the obvious when we

sat down at the dinner table. The chicken, the salad, and the mashed potatoes. I'd see my wife, looking like she was always running behind schedule. And the kids with a thousand stories of things happening at school. That was what was in front of me. That's what I saw.

"But last night I saw from my heart," continued Peter, struggling to hold back his emotions. "I looked around that table and saw something quite different. For the first time, I saw this precious moment where the minds, bodies, and souls of our family were gathered together to break bread and be nourished. There was so much more there than just the food. There were lives filled with potential for good. We were there to help each other, to love each other, to care for each other."

Peter paused as he relived that special moment in his mind. "And the children even got into an argument with their mother. But instead of driving me up the wall, that argument was different. Or at least I saw it differently. It seemed to be a natural expression of love toward each other, a way of saying, 'I care.' "

Spiritual eyes help us *see* the high value of what is simple and readily available in our lives in spite of the circumstances in which we may find ourselves.

"I awoke from my surgery," said Pontea, "and there in my room was my husband. He was holding our little daughter up on the hospital bed. And she was holding my finger. Her big dark eyes looked at me, and she smiled as she said, 'I love you, Mommy.' It was such a precious moment. Now, since my cancer, I see so much more of life."

This level of awareness brings, to the person who will see, a vastly different experience of illness and of life. There are miraculous moments in our lives right now—every day. We just need to see them.

## AN IMPORTANT THING YOU CAN DO

Tonight, or the next time you are together with family or friends, take a few moments to see life in this new light. Ask yourself, "What do these people really mean to me?" This could do more for your well-being than the most powerful medicine.

# #45

## VALUE PERSONAL SPIRITUAL GROWTH

Too many people equate victory over cancer with a doctor's report that says "This patient is clinically free of cancer." I understand that desire, I share that desire, and, in fact, my records state exactly that. I wish you the same. But that is not the most important part of the journey through cancer.

For the thinking person, the cancer journey quickly evolves into a spiritual quest. Survivors are nearly unanimous on this issue. The real triumph over cancer is realized in the nurturing of personal spiritual growth.

Some people say, "I'll settle for a cure and just get my life back to normal." Don't settle for that! After your experience with cancer, things will never be the same again. You don't want things to get back to normal. You want a new and better life. That life comes in the form of personal spiritual growth.

Cancer has pounded you with a million hammer blows. But you have the last word as to how those blows will shape you. William James, the great psychologist and philosopher, declared that his generation's most important discovery was that human beings, by changing their inner attitudes of mind, could change the outer aspects of their lives. I believe the hammer blows of cancer, or of any difficult problem, can be used to help us grow spiritually. And by doing the work of wellness, making personal spiritual growth our aim, I believe we can use cancer to shape us into wonderfully different people. *Cancer can change attitudes and transform our lives.*

Think of personal spiritual growth as a natural extension of your wellness journey. You are going to devote time and energy to getting better. You'll look within to uncover and develop your own practice of gratitude, forgiveness, unconditional love, and more. This is the high and rewarding call of the work of wellness.

Cynicism has no place here. You cannot climb the spiritual mountain by thinking downhill thoughts. If you feel that life is filled with despair, that it is gloomy and hopeless, that spiritual growth is impossible for you, it is because *you* are gloomy and hopeless. You must change your mind to change your spirit. If you do, you will change your inner world, which will in turn change your outer world. This is powerful healing.

Associate with men and women who are walking the spiritual path. Your change can be advanced by meeting and mingling with those who have a spiritual vision. Be inspired by our great spiritual ancestors from all the ages.

And finally, pray. Don't beg or plead. Be still and prayerfully listen to the God of your understanding. Personal spiritual growth can be most effectively accomplished through the power of prayer. Remember, all things *are* possible.

### AN IMPORTANT THING YOU CAN DO

In your wellness workbook, record one quality of spiritual growth, such as forgiveness, that you would like to practice today. Start by making a commitment to practice that quality for just one hour. Then extend the time. Keep this as your central goal, your main objective. Opportunities for practice will present themselves every moment of the day. You just have to see them.

# #46

## DISCOVER
## YOUR
## EMOTIONAL
## STYLE

By now you know that emotions have a central role in wellness. One of the most energy-charged emotions is anger. Anger is generally short-lived, a sudden emotion over a single event. It's a feeling with which all of us are familiar. Anger is natural. We express it. It's human.

Resentment wears a mask. It looks like anger but it is actually *unresolved* anger, emotions, and feelings that we cling to. While anger is expressed and forgotten, resentment is not forgotten. With resentment, we impose stress on ourselves by reliving the anger in our minds. Each time we recall the event, our negative feelings are re-experienced. We feel the stress and conflict at the time of the event, and we rehearse the stress with each memory. This practice works powerfully against our wellness.

Some people carry past resentments with them for years. I'm sure you've heard people recall in great detail childhood experiences that caused them sorrow. Maybe it was a lack of parental love. Others talk about rejection by a spouse or a teacher. Or maybe it was a business deal that went bad. The points of anger, now turned to smoldering embers of resentment, are endless.

Emotions themselves are not inherently bad. Don't judge whether you are a good or bad person based on your emotional responses. The truth is, it's okay to be angry at times. Check yourself. Observe your emotional reactions. Feel the anger and express it. Don't cling to it. That's what plants the seed for the deadly emotion, resentment.

How do we get around this anger/resentment trap? Simple. Learn to focus on the *event*, not the emotions. What actually provoked you? This will get you beyond the emotional response to the conflict at the center of the problem. It will even set the process of resolution in motion.

This increased awareness is powerful! If we will just reflect on the event, we will often discover that we perceived the "provoker"—be it a person, event, or condition—with fear. We were the ones who were fearful that our person, property, or pride was under attack. Therefore, the deeper emotion we are dealing with is fear, not anger or resentment.

This is a profound discovery of highest importance, one that affects us on every level of our lives. It's fear we are dealing with, our own fear, *something that is under our control.* If we allow that fear to become obsessive, it will affect us biochemically as the body harbors our resentments. Suddenly we realize that our negative emotions carry a big price—to the point of depressing our immune systems at the very time we need them to function at their peak.

Becoming keenly aware of our emotions and observing the situations that prompt them allows us to rethink our fear-based perception that we are under siege. Instead of perceiving fear, try to understand the situation in the light of compassion. This is a new and miraculous emotional response, one that begins to dissolve resentments and heal us on many levels.

Impossible? Not at all! Like it or not, the other person, the situation, the doctor, God—none of those is responsible for making us angry. We make ourselves angry. And we can choose to replace resentment with positive and compassionate responses.

Potent energy like anger can be expressed and dismissed. That's healthy. But to see life constantly through the lens of fear, always perceiving events as a threat, consistently responding with anger and clinging to past hurts, reliving and rehearsing the poisonous negative emotions as we recall the events, cripples us with resentment. This has no place in the wellness journey.

### AN IMPORTANT THING YOU CAN DO

Discover your personal emotional style. Be an objective observer over the next week. When an upset occurs, identify your emotional response in one of three terms: denial, repression, or overreaction.

Record the upsetting event in your wellness notebook. Then write down your emotional response based on one of three categories: "I *denied* that there was any problem"; "I *repressed* my emotions when I really wanted to tell that S.O.B. off"; or "I went crazy and *overreacted*, way out of proportion to the whole event."

If you do this exercise consistently, you'll become a skilled observer of your own emotional stance toward life. Reactions and emotions that were once automatic will now come under your control. This knowledge will become a major contributor to your total well-being, even saving your immune system from the biochemical ravages of negative emotions.

# #47

# MAKE
# FORGIVENESS
# A HABIT

Do you want to free all your energy to heal? Forgive!

Forgiveness is wellness work that brings with it huge rewards. Forgiveness takes our newfound awareness of the important relationships in our lives and our deeper understanding of our emotional style and gives us the peace and serenity we need for healing. That is a big promise. Forgiveness can deliver.

Forgiveness is the lost key to wellness. Forgiveness is the singular technique by which our thoughts and perceptions are changed, transforming the harmful effects of fear to the healing reality of love. Altering our focus from fear to love while traveling the cancer journey helps us change what can be changed and allows us to make peace with the rest. This is healing of the highest order.

Forgiveness starts by letting ourselves off the hook. We hold so many resentments against ourselves and don't let go easily. In the quiet moments we judge ourselves harshly. Now, like never before, is the time in your life to release that self-condemnation. The only way is through self-forgiveness.

I believe many cancer patients tend to think of themselves as not worthy on a deep level. That is such a deadly and false belief. Yes, we may have done something undesirable, but that is our behavior and does not equate with being a bad person. This false perception is the cause of much pain and works against our well-being.

Our perceptions of others can also create a battleground of emotional turmoil. It is so easy to judge others. Judgmental behavior tears at the fabric of relationships and kindles the fires of resentment. Cancer is, among other things, an opportunity to learn and practice the difference between acceptance and approval. All of us have imperfect natures. Accept that as fact. All of us exhibit behaviors that don't match our potential. Accept that as fact. We can accept imperfection without having to approve of it. Not everything will exactly meet our expectations. Forgiving ourselves and others is at the heart of practicing the difference between acceptance and approval.

Forgiveness has two levels. The first is the most obvious. There is an event: Someone is wronged, and that behavior needs to be forgiven. When we can say, "I forgive myself for _____," or "I forgive _____ (another) for _____," we have started on the forgiveness journey.

The second level of forgiveness changes our perception of what happened. Yes, an event occurred. But the real problem starts when we begin to *judge* what happened, when we start to label ourselves or the other person as bad, hurtful, mean, stupid, or some other less-than-kind term. We perceived the event as unfavorable; the event didn't meet our approval; we judged it. Understand how the negative cycle perpetuates itself.

The alternative? Acceptance. Accept others. Accept ourselves. Accept life. This is a far better way to live. People who are or believe themselves to be near death often come to the realization that forgiveness heals. Feuds, differences, and deep hurts suddenly seem less important at this time. I can understand. I had to learn this lesson myself. Hundreds, even thousands of patients have shared similar stories.

Marilyn, who had ovarian cancer, felt terribly ill at ease when her mother and father visited her. Marilyn and her mother would make noble efforts to get along with each other, but they seldom succeeded fully. Old patterns of attack and defense were constantly cropping up between them. Child care, cooking, homemaking, religion—the particulars didn't seem to matter. Her mother wanted a more conservative daughter. Marilyn wanted a more enlightened mother.

"It was driving me crazy," said Marilyn. "During her last visit, I was ready to throw her out. But then it occurred to me, God isn't looking at my mother and thinking, 'Mildred is such a bitch.' How could I pretend to want to get along with my mother if I was so consumed by my judgment of her errors? I had to practice acceptance and get off my fixation with approval.

"So I said to myself, 'I'll try this for an afternoon. I'll focus on acceptance and give up approval.' From that moment, the situation and the relationship started to shift. As I was more accepting of her, she became more accepting of me. We're a long way from best buddies," conceded Marilyn, "but there is a growing bond between us."

The amazing payoff of forgiveness is that so many people get well after extending forgiveness! Lives are certainly made better and many are made longer. But it strikes me that if one is willing to forgive during the last moments of life, why not do it earlier? Like right now?

How often do we need to forgive? Always. Don't drag the memories of past hurts and mistakes into your present moments. Nothing from the past is important enough to allow it to pollute your present. Family, relationships, acceptance, understanding, and compassion are much more important than holding on to the past at the expense of present-moment wellness. Forgive. You'll change your life!

## AN IMPORTANT THING YOU CAN DO

Choose one hurt or mistake and forgive everyone concerned with it. Say, out loud, "(name), I totally and completely forgive you." Mean it. Now feel the warmth of forgiveness. Its called freedom—and wellness! Choose to forgive one person each day.

# #48

---

## EXUDE
## GRATITUDE

Have you expressed your thankfulness today? We all have so many blessings to appreciate every day of our lives. But most of us have to consciously practice being grateful.

Even with cancer, even in the middle of treatment, even in your darkest hours, be thankful for all you do have. For life, for love, for family, for friends, for the awesome beauty of nature, for the presence of God, for all these things and more, be thankful. Thousands of survivors are convinced that there is a biochemical correlative to such an attitude. Their bodies respond.

With this attitude of gratitude, see yourself as a guest who is only visiting here on earth. All that you have is not really yours, it is a gracious gift from your host that you are privileged to use during your stay. Even your health, no matter what the state, is another of those gifts. Aren't we fortunate to experience this brief moment in time that we are guests here?

Jill lay near death in a small rural Nebraska hospital after being told she was "filled" with cancer and that it was inoperable. Mired in despair and self-pity, she could see nothing to be thankful for. "I was divorced, my two children were grown and lived in different parts of the country, I had a job I hated, my life seemed miserable.

"But one night I looked out of my hospital window to see a deep dark sky that was filled with stars. I shut off all the lights in my room and just gazed at that sky for what must have been hours. I started to ask a lot of questions: What is this huge universe about? What is my place in it? Why am I sick? I can't say I got a lot of answers. But I did get a different perspective.

"I became thankful," continued Jill, "grateful just for being a part of this huge and wonderful world. I realized that in my fifty-plus years, I had been able to experience so much. The marvel of having given birth to two other lives—what a miracle! The beauty of the country where I feel such strong roots—I was so grateful to live here rather than in a city. The deep friendship I had with my sister—I was so thankful for her love. That night at the window changed my whole perspective on my problems."

Like Jill, we can capture the wellness that derives from gratitude. But much of the cancer journey seems to stand in the way of doing so. We're so busy with appointments and treatments and other things that we lose our perspective. We tend to look at the cancer journey as a long series of negatives. There seems to be nothing to be thankful for about this situation. This is faulty thinking. There is much to be thankful for.

Gratitude transforms the very experience of illness and of life. Gratitude is one component of viewing the world with spiritual eyes. See beyond the day-to-day experiences that seem so all-consuming. Treasure the wonder of life. Become aware of your "guest status" in this brief moment in time that we visit the earth. Be thankful. It heals.

AN IMPORTANT THING YOU CAN DO

It's time for another new page in your wellness notebook. Label the page *What I am thankful for today.* You may want to divide the page into three columns: *People*, *Places*, and *Things*. Be thankful for all the gifts. And express your thanks.

# #49

# PRACTICE
# UNCONDITIONAL
# LOVING

Loving heals. Even though there may be times when we are lost in the abyss of our physical maladies or buried in the agony of our emotional "awfulizing," with each moment comes a new opportunity to choose loving. This is a decision, a personal choice. And this choice truly heals.

Loving, without conditions, means we don't have to wait for the medical-test results, the doctor's assurances, the elusive remission, or the hoped-for cure. We can choose to love now, this moment. And the next moment. And then we choose again. We always have that choice, regardless of the circumstances.

The crippling fears surrounding cancer are actually the absence of love. It's like darkness that is merely the absence of light. You don't solve a problem of darkness by yelling at it or trying to strike at it. If you want to get rid of the darkness, you turn on a light. So it is with fear. You don't fight it. You replace fear with love.

I prefer the word *loving*. It denotes the *action* necessary to bring the idea of love to life. Love is not loving until it is *enacted*, until it is *given*. This means choosing to exercise our benevolence and compassion to ourselves and others in this moment despite any circumstance, including the circumstance of cancer.

This is a profound and radical call, not some live-with-loving-feelings suggestion. Loving is more than a thin veneer. Loving is an act of heroism and courage of the highest order. But don't seek or even expect accolades. Unconditional loving is usually not a choice surrounded by pomp and circumstance. Most often it has to do with small choices: "How do I choose to respond to this information?" "Should I focus on the positive?" "Would eating this be in my best interests?" "Would exercising help my total well-being?" "How can I help another person?" "How can I love myself?"

The conditions and circumstances alone may not warrant loving. Taken by themselves, the conditions may elicit despair. But this is where choice comes in. We can take the loving action anyway! Invariably, the result is a renewed sense of hope that results in a strong biochemical "live" signal to our body, mind, and spirit.

Loving must start with self-loving. You can hope to know wellness only from a position of personal emotional and spiritual strength. Self-loving is the wellspring of this vital force. Affirm your great value; cancer does not detract from that. Self-loving is the real starting point of recovery for many patients.

Does loving seem too difficult a task? Does your mind say that you can never be at peace until the cancer is gone? Do you feel that a total and complete physical cure is the only acceptable answer? Does it seem impossible to love with the sword of cancer balancing precariously over your head? Love anyway. For if you love, you will be healed on the highest level.

Loving is the first and last word in healing, the great balm that quiets stress, the only real "magic bullet" against cancer, and the strongest vaccine to combat malignancy.

Our greatest enemy is not the fear of disease but the torment of despair. Unconditional loving is the healer. And the first object of your unconditional loving is *you!*

### AN IMPORTANT THING YOU CAN DO

It is decision time. Decide to practice unconditional loving for the next hour. And the next hour ... and the next ...

# #50

# SHARE
# THIS
# HOPE

Now that you've invested time reading this book and following at least some of the steps, you're aware that there is much you can do to improve your wellness. Your choices and actions do make an enormous difference. And, in partnership with your medical team, you are on the pathway to healing.

But most people don't know these truths. Or if they do, they have only a vague acquaintance with the principles, not a working knowledge. This is not enough.

Share this hope. Tell others who have been diagnosed with cancer about these ideas. Encourage one another. Make it your new priority to walk the path of wellness with someone else. This has the cumulative effect of helping yourself while helping another. Through your decision to serve, two get well. Make that decision today.

And write to us. We have a free newsletter for you, plus a variety of helpful wellness resources. You have a caring partner in your journey:

The Cancer Conquerors Foundation
P.O. Box 238
Hershey, PA 17033

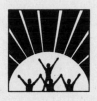

# EPILOGUE

# YOU
# HAVE
# A FUTURE

While cancer is certainly a serious physical illness, anyone who has fought the battle knows that it is as much a psychological and spiritual battle as a physical one. And they know what a meaningful difference the mind and spirit make.

Tap deeply into the mental and spiritual assets you have been given. Understand the truth and power behind them. And use illness as an opportunity for personal growth. That may seem beyond the scope of your current thinking. But believe that it can be accomplished. Illness has been the pathway for millions of people to discover an even better life than they ever dreamed possible. Illness can be your wake-up call, a chance to experience the life you may have been forced to put on hold.

No matter how much time you think you may have to live, make the decision to live today fully alive! Make the profound choices to forgive and to love. This leads to a full life and, as thousands of us believe, a longer life as well.

Let this illness be your new beginning. Choose this moment to be well, to the fullest extent. A happy future can be yours. Personal choice and present-moment spiritual living are truly the most important things you can do when the doctor says, "It's cancer."

# SURVEY
## ON CANCER
## AND RECOVERY

Your help is needed. If you are eighteen years of age or older, please take a few moments to answer the following questions. Please use a separate sheet of paper. You need not include your name.

The purpose of this survey is to learn in greater depth how people cope with cancer. Your experiences could be of tremendous help to others who are confronting the illness.

The combined responses of this questionnaire will be published. However, no respondent will be identified by name without prior written permission. All answers to the questions are voluntary. If you do not want to answer a question, feel free to skip it and go on to the next one.

1. Describe your type of cancer, the month and year of initial diagnosis and recurrence, if applicable, and the recommended treatment program(s). Did you obtain a second opinion? Were you treated by a board-certified oncologist?
2. What was the most difficult part, physically, emotionally, and spiritually? Be specific. Include as many details as possible.

3. How did your cancer affect your family, including spouse, children, and/or parents? Who was the most helpful? Least helpful? Why?

4. How has cancer affected your faith? How has your faith affected your cancer?

5. In addition to medical doctors, have you sought professional help from a psychologist, a member of the clergy, and/or others? Did you use nontraditional treatment? If so, what? How would you rate the effectiveness of the help, including your medical team?

6. How have your friends responded to your cancer?

7. Have you attended a cancer support group? If yes, who was the sponsor? How often do you attend? How would you rate the effectiveness of the help?

8. Has cancer changed the fundamental values by which you live your life? If so, in what ways?

9. What advice do you have for someone who is confronting a cancer diagnosis?

10. Was this book helpful to you? What was most helpful? Least helpful?

Please mail your response to this survey to:
Survey on Cancer and Recovery
The Cancer Conquerors Foundation
P.O. Box 238
Hershey, PA 17033

# ABOUT
# THE AUTHOR

GREG ANDERSON is living proof that there is much one can do to help oneself in the cancer journey. Diagnosed with metastasized lung cancer in 1984, he was given only thirty days to live. Refusing to accept the hopelessness of this prognosis, he went searching for people who had lived when their doctors had told them they were "supposed" to die. His findings, from interviews with hundreds of survivors, form the principles and action points of this powerful and hope-filled book.

In 1985 Greg started the Cancer Conquerors Foundation, an organization that provides training and support for implementing body/mind/spirit principles. Services include seminars, workshops, support groups. audiovisual programs, self-assessment tools, and a free newsletter, "Creating Wellness."

The Anderson family lives in the Los Angeles area. Greg and his wife, Linda, are the parents of one daughter, Erica. Prior to his illness, Greg was vice-president and executive director of the Robert Schuller Institute, located at the Crystal Cathedral in Garden Grove, California. He is also the author of two inspirational best sellers, *The Cancer Conqueror* and *The Triumphant Patient*. Today he travels extensively to speak and conduct workshops, sharing his experience and techniques.

# BECOME A MEMBER OF...

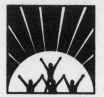

T H E
# CANCER
# CONQUERORS
F O U N D A T I O N